Gotcha Covered:
A Legacy of Service and Protection

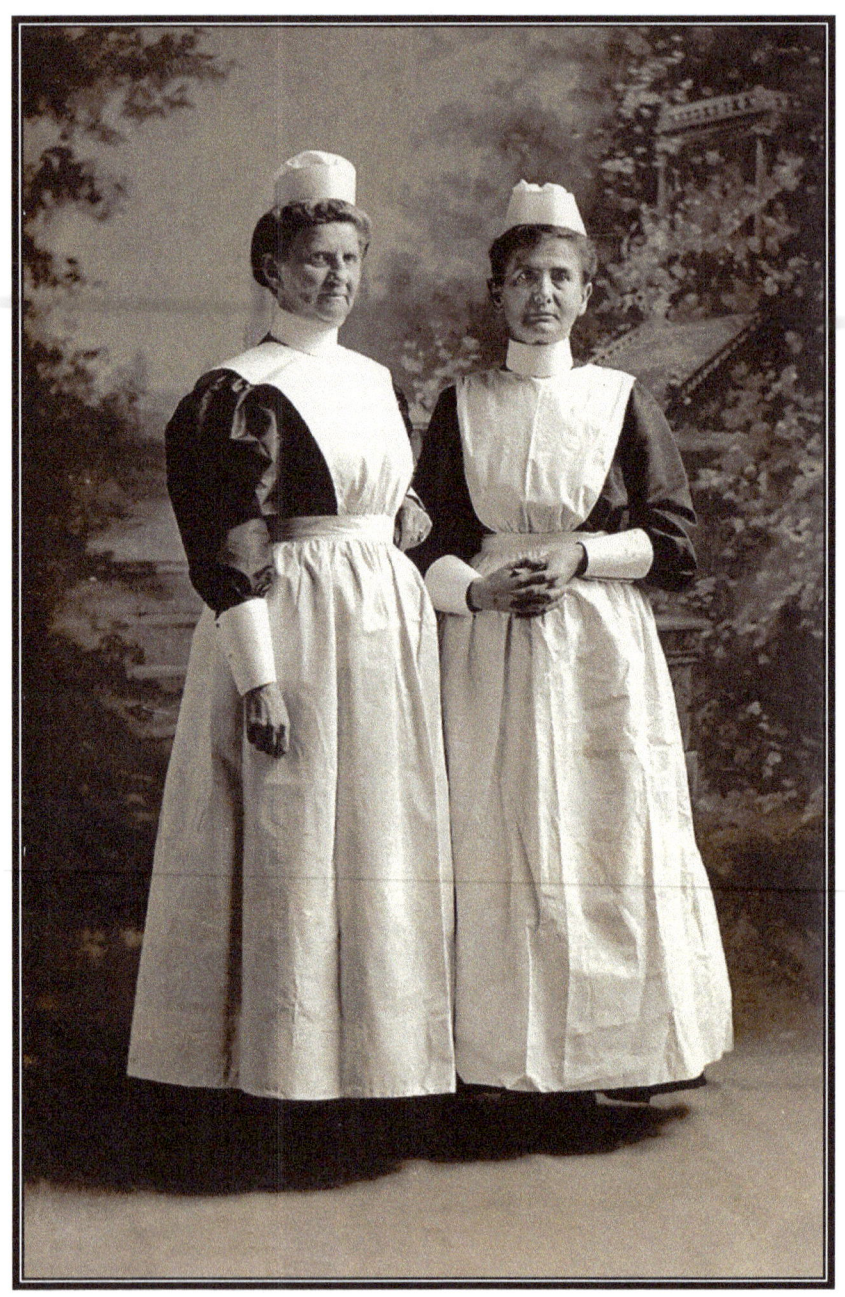

© Zwerdling Nursing Archives, used with permission.

Gotcha Covered:
A Legacy of Service and Protection

An Anthology of The Nurses' Apron Partnership

Edited by Ginger T. Manley
Foreword by Virginia Trotter Betts

PUBLISHED BY WESTVIEW, INC., NASHVILLE, TN

GOTCHA COVERED: A LEGACY OF SERVICE AND PROTECTION

PUBLISHED BY WESTVIEW, INC.
P.O. Box 210183
Nashville, Tennessee 37221
www.publishedbywestview.com

© 2009 Ginger T. Manley
All rights reserved, including the right to reproduction in whole or in part in any form.
ISBN Case laminate: 978-1-935271-23-9; ISBN Perfect bound: 978-1-935271-35-2

Credits:

The front cover design is an adaptation of an original watercolor by Maxine Arnold Dalton and is used with her permission.

The photographs of aprons in this book were commissioned and were taken by Rod Daniel, unless otherwise noted. They are © 2009 Ginger Manley

The archival images of nurse postcards are © Zwerdling Nursing Archives and are used with permission of Michael Zwerdling. www.nursepostcard.com. The images were previously published in *Postcards of Nursing: A Worldwide Tribute* (Lippincott Williams & Wilkins, 2004)

The reproduction of the vintage McCall pattern #1279 is © 1946 McCall Patterns and is used with permission of McCall/ Butterick Vogue Pattern Company.

The G.E. print advertisement originally appeared in the March, 1952, *Better Homes and Gardens* and is © 1952 General Electric Company, used with permission.

The Tappan ad is reproduced courtesy of Electrolux. It originally appeared in the March, 1952 *Better Homes and Gardens*.

The two SafeBabies infant emergency evacuation aprons illustrations are used with permission of International Health Resources, www.safebabiesaprons.com.

The image of Mary Jo Reimer in South Africa was photographed by Nicole Itano and is used with her permission. It previously appeared in *Christian Science Monitor*, Oct. 17, 2001.

The images of dolls dressed as nursing students were photographed by Doug Sturgeon and are © 2008 Vanderbilt University School of Nursing, used with permission.

The dogwood image was photographed by Tom Wortham and is used with his permission.

The images of R.N's in Kenya were photgraphed by Stacey Irvin and are used with her permission.

The hand drawn artwork was submitted and is used with permission of the artists: Hannah Cozzolino, Morgan Cozzolino, and Taylor Politan.

The TNAP graphics were commissioned and were created by Stacey Irvin.

"Kitchen Art Collage" by Sally Reinhart Crowe is used with permission.

"Benn Art Card" by Patricia Vuleta Spence Benn is used with permission.

All other photographs were submitted by the authors.

Back cover photograph of Susan Kaburu was submitted and is used with Kaburu's permission.

Printed in the United States of America on acid free paper
www.thenursesapronpartnership.com

In memory of

Alice Trundle

and in honor of her sister

Katherine Maloney

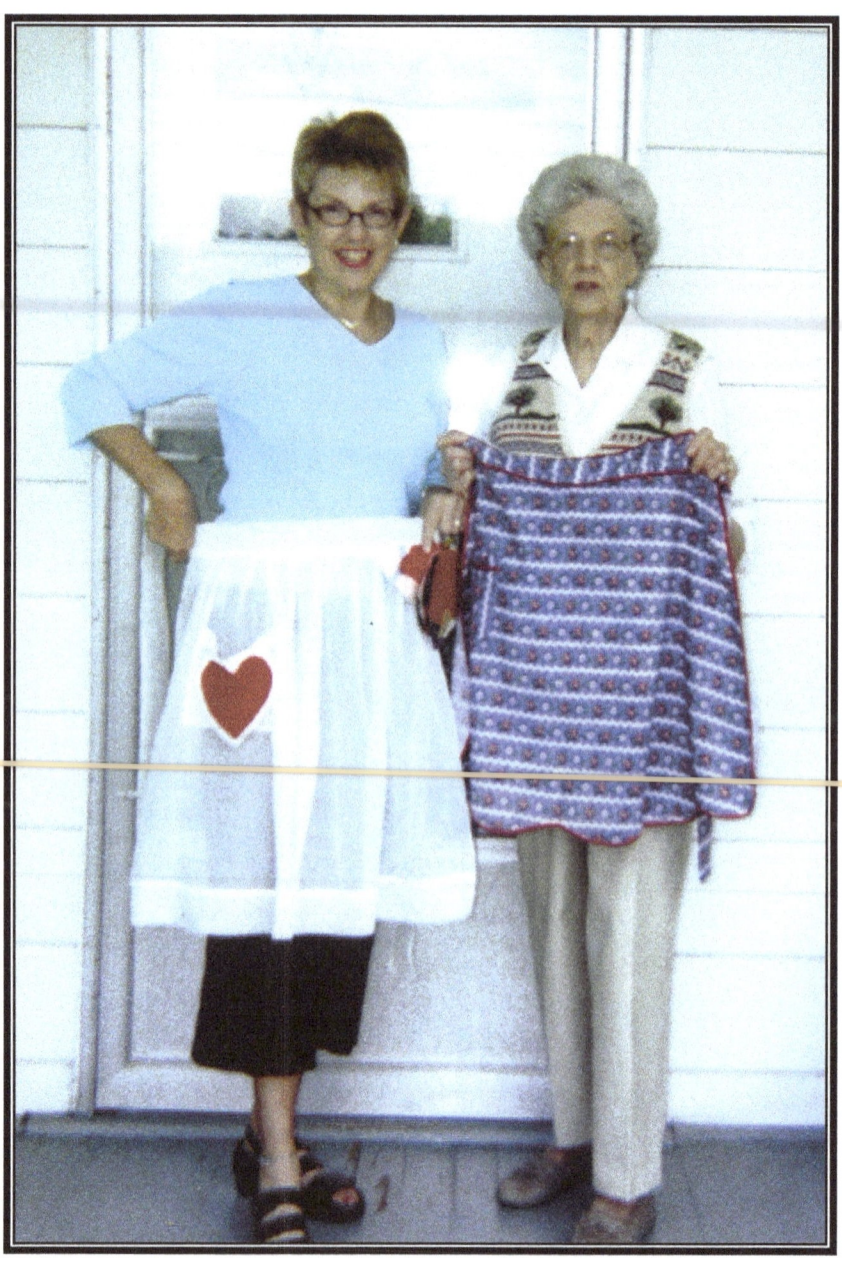

Author Ginger Manley and her Aunt Katherine Maloney, the original owner of most of the aprons in this book

*When I talk about aprons, it's one thing,
but when you can touch them, it becomes not just a basket of aprons,
or a clothesline of aprons,
but a clothesline of stories.*

EllynAnne Geisel

The Nurses' Apron Partnership

All royalties from the sale of *Gotcha Covered: A Legacy of Service and Protection* go to Burning Bush, Inc., a 501(c)3 nonprofit corporation.

If you would like to support the work of Burning Bush, Inc. directly, please visit www.burningbushkenya.org. You may also contribute directly at:

    Burning Bush, Inc.
    1557 Harding Place
    Nashville, TN 37215

To learn more about The Nurses' Apron Partnership and our ongoing efforts in funding micro-credit loans for Kenyan RN's through Burning Bush, Inc., please visit www.thenursesapronpartnership.com

Gotcha Covered: A Legacy of Service and Protection can be purchased online at
http://www.publishedbywestview.com/gotchacovered.html
and in select retail stores.

For credit card or check orders, contact:

Published by Westview, Inc.
8120 Sawyer Brown Road, Suite 107
P.O. Box 210183
Nashville, Tennessee 37221
phone (615) 646 6134
fax   (615) 662 0946

Contents

FOREWORD xiii
    Virginia Trotter Betts

PREFACE xv

INTRODUCTION xvii

PART ONE: *Aprons as Symbols of Healing* 1

    Introduction by Ginger T. Manley 3

        IN OUR VOICES: THE LEGACY OF NURSING 7

            Kathleen L. Wolff 9
            Marilyn Bache Sonnenberg 11
            Karen L. Starr 13
            Joan Crosland Chapman Sughrue 15
            Mary Jo Reimer 17
            Barbara Siddens Vinson 21
            Judith B. Collins 23
            Sara Jeanne Wells 27
            Amanda Taylor Pendley 29
            Rebekah Nesbitt 33
            Susan Kaburu 35
            Virginia M. George 37
            Brooke Faught 39
            Cindy Fielder Diamond 41

PART TWO: *Aprons as Symbols of Identity and Service* 43

    Introduction by Ginger T. Manley 45

Gotcha Covered: A Legacy of Service and Protection

Identity Legacies: 53

Apron Remembrances 55
Carol Etherington

Pressing Matters 57
Marti Mueller Daniel

Apron Tribute 61
Mary Gresham Buchanan Barr

My Apron, My Self 65
Ginger T. Manley

Judge A Woman By Her Apron! Not! 69
Diane Carlson Evans

The Abandoned Apron 73
Maxine Arnold Dalton

Service Legacies: 77

An Apron Of Service 79
Krista Koleas

The Word: Hospitality 81
Margaret Kuehnle Fulton

Celebrate Life 83
Poppy Pickering Buchanan

Part Three: *Aprons as Symbols of Comfort* 85

Introduction by Ginger T. Manley 87

Kitchen Legacies: 89

Kitchen Art 91
Sally Reinhart Crowe

Little Apron 93
Sharron Stewart Burch

Look For Us In The Kitchen 95
Linda Schlesinger Mabry

THE APRON 99
    Donna Maddox
COMING OF AGE ONE MONTH BEFORE THANKSGIVING 101
    Sally Yeagley
MY GRANDMA'S KITCHEN 105
    Lisa Fournace

MOTHERING LEGACIES: 107

APRON CARD 109
    Patricia Vuleta Spence Benn
THE EVERYDAY APRON 111
    Linda Scott Herzfeld
MOM 113
    Sharon Adkins
APRONS 115
    Beverly Byram
TEXANNA JONES 117
    Kathleen S. Lewis
A CLOUD OF LAVENDER-BLUE 121
    Dianne Horton Wood
MY APRON MEMORIES 123
    Marceleen Rodes Alford
GRANDMA'S APRONS 125
    Sue Wilson
APRON IMAGES 127
    Jennie Maddra Fleshood

GENERATIONAL LEGACIES: 129

THE APRON INTERVIEW 131
    Marilyn Hobbs McAtee
APRON MEMORIES 135
    Libby Dayani
APRONS . . . TIES . . . TRADITIONS . . . CHANGES . . . GENERATIONS 139
    Charlotte Richardson Norwood

PART FOUR: *Aprons as Symbols of Imagination and Creativity* 141

   Introduction by Ginger T. Manley 143

      FICTION: 147

         NOTHIN' SAYS LOVIN' 149
           Suzanne Hopkins Blievernicht
         THE WORRY APRON 157
           Carol E. Dixon
         THE GREEN APRON 163
           Ellen E. McGeady
         MONTANA MEMORIES 169
           Judy Tincher Monaco
         THE REMNANT 171
           Frances McGaughy Edwards

      NONFICTION: 173

         THE WEDDING APRON 175
           Lydia Luttrell Grubb
         A POCKET SURPRISE 179
           Myra Wilson Willey
         THE HAPPY CHILDHOOD OF GRANDMA IDA GILMORE 181
           Louise Colln

THE NURSES' APRON PARTNERSHIP 185
   Ginger T. Manley

ACKNOWLEDGMENTS 187

BIBLIOGRAPHY AND REFERENCES 191

LIST OF CONTRIBUTORS 199

PHOTOGRAPHIC AND ILLUSTRATION CREDITS 207

Foreword

At least half the nurses who contributed to this anthology have been colleagues, classmates, or students of mine, but until I read their contributions to this book, I would never have thought of them as *apron people*. I am certainly not much of an apron person myself. Rather, I have spent most of my professional life championing the causes of women, nurses, and health care throughout Tennessee and the nation, by way of Washington, D.C.

The Tennessee Nurses' Association, the American Nurses' Association, the U.S. Department of Health & Human Services, and now the Tennessee Department of Mental Health & Developmental Disabilities have been my points of passionate, professional involvement—along with Vanderbilt University and University of Tennessee Health Sciences Center. I am not a domestic diva in the least—with or without an apron—but then, come to think of it, neither are many of the nurses I know who contributed to this book. So I was intrigued to know how aprons—that humblest of garments and completely missing from my wardrobe—came to be entwined with the lives of these forty-nine nurses. And even more so, how the combined efforts of the nurses could foster a grassroots effort to reach out to nurse colleagues in Kenya.

I discovered that every one of the nurses had been influenced, in some way, by an apron or by someone in their lives who wore an apron. I, like them, was shaped by wonderful women wearing aprons—and pantsuits and uniforms. Growing up in East Tennessee, I was nurtured by a grandmother who was never without her apron. She raised nine children, including my father. Her home was filled with noise, laughter, and an incredible aroma of fabulous food. Today, my own family enjoys—on rare occasions—delicious meals made from her recipes.

The vintage aprons that inspired this book, and ultimately inspired the outreach program of The Nurses' Apron Partnership, came from another little community in East Tennessee very close to my hometown. While I do not have any cherished aprons from my mother, grandmother, or aunts, I do have apron memories. My life has been so influenced by my mother, Alice Trotter, and my aunt, Mary Emily Trotter, both public health nurses who were committed to their work and their profession. Many times, they threw an apron over their blue uniforms to cook for family and friends, and then dashed off to TNA or TPHA meetings. Neither of them encouraged me to become a nurse, but they were thrilled when I did.

Gotcha Covered: A Legacy of Service and Protection tells the story of aprons and of nurses. Aprons and nurses share an essential nature—both tend to be invisible and undervalued. I am so pleased to be joining with my colleagues, in this book and worldwide, to bring more visibility to the essentiality of nursing through the metaphor of the apron, and in doing so, to support the efforts of The Nurses' Apron Partnership.

Virginia Trotter Betts, MSN, JD, FAAN
Commissioner, Tennessee Department of Mental Health & Developmental Disabilities
Past President, American and Tennessee Nurses' Associations
Nashville, TN
May 2009

Preface

We were seated in the most remote booth in the busy, upscale restaurant near the university where I had been his student almost fifty years before. I arrived before him for our meeting and requested to be seated where there would be the least amount of background noise. In freshman English in 1962, most of the women students had occupied the front row whenever possible, leaning forward to hear the voice of this most respected young professor. In 2008, I wore hearing aids, and again I leaned forward, this time straining to hear his familiar, soft, and occasionally muffled voice with its pronounced Southern accent.

I was pretty sure he didn't really get it. We had been conversing about the aprons for almost ninety minutes while lunch was ordered, served, and eaten. In between bites of tilapia and sips of unsweetened tea, I answered his questions and gave him my best shot at explaining the story of the aprons—complete with the research we had done that linked aprons to feminism, nursing, and heartfelt emotions. I told him we concluded that aprons were vehicles for connections of many kinds, but especially as metaphors for identity, for comfort, for healing, and for imagination. We discussed the role of academic women and feminist research and writing, and pondered whether his female counterparts in the Department of English would feel any attraction for these aprons. He urged me to be relentless in separating the truly wonderful pieces from the just so-so pieces, and we considered how and where to push for publication. So I knew he was being, in every sense, the teacher and mentor I needed to help take this work from a pile of stories in a folder to a robust manuscript begging to be devoured by readers worldwide. But he didn't really get it.

Then, as he was settling up the bill with the twenty-something server who had been attending us, he looked up at her and asked, "Do you wear an apron at home?"

She paused, a look of confusion on her face.

He smiled. "That's not a come-on."

Pointing in my direction, he told her, "We've just been discussing aprons and I wondered if after taking off your serving apron here . . . when you go home, do you ever wear an apron there?"

Thinking she might still be confused, or perhaps this had crossed a personal boundary for her, I said, "I'm writing a book about aprons."

She smiled broadly.

He opened the folder, which contained some of the manuscript, and pulled out the photographs of the aprons.

"Look." He pointed. "Like these. Do you ever wear an apron in your own kitchen?"

She fingered through the apron photos, lingering to absorb the image of several, and then she replied, "No, I don't have an apron at home. I almost never cook—I eat take-out or just micro something. But some of my friends cook and they have aprons."

She looked back at the apron photos now splayed across the table, touching a couple of them gently with her index finger. Her face softened and her eyes began to shine. She stood back from the table and gained about an inch in height. Then cocking her head to the left, she moved her hands to either side of her waist and began to pantomime putting on an apron, drawing the ties behind her and making a bow with the imaginary apron strings.

"If I had an apron like one of these, I'd put it on and . . . I could become anyone—my grandmother, anyone. It would be way-cool!"

I looked at my lunch companion and he was transfixed. As he turned his gaze back to me and the young woman began clearing away the rest of the lunch dishes, he smiled.

"That is the first paragraph of your book," he said.

Ginger T. Manley

INTRODUCTION

If we can no longer understand the language, the few remaining old aprons will remain mute.
                                                            Avis Smith, *The Language of Aprons: Signifiers of Femininity*

When several discrete entities, having parts in common, are arranged so they overlap each other in order to show what part or parts they share, the graphic image of such an arrangement is called a Venn diagram. This book is like a Venn diagram, where each of three independent circles—feminism, aprons, and the profession of nursing—overlap in a central area. It is from that central convergence—and sometimes the divergence—that the soul and spirit of this book emerges.

The term *feminism* dates from the late 1890s and involves theory, policies, movements, and activities that advocate equality for women, including women's rights. There are several competing schools of thought about feminism—the white, western, middle-class view; the African-American view; and the Third World view. The following summary is very general, reflecting mostly the Anglo-North American, white experience.

Feminism in the United States is divided into four phases or waves. The first phase began in the early eighteen hundreds, when females pushed for ownership and inheritance rights, and later when women began to lobby for voting rights equal to those granted men in 1870. Passage of the Nineteenth Amendment to the Constitution in 1919 is generally regarded as the end of first-wave feminism. The second wave of feminism began around 1960, and extended through the 1970s and 1980s. During this time, women were struggling for workplace, reproductive, and educational equality and rights. The third wave extended from the 1990s until the end of the twentieth century, when women were reevaluating their recently won, equal roles in society, and integrating these with the more traditional roles of parent and homemaker. The fourth wave of feminism, roughly tied to the events of September 11, 2001, is about wisdom—about transforming the experiences of life's journey into meaningful events, through spiritually informed activism. Women worldwide have responded to this time by using their wisdom to help heal something—perhaps the divisions between selves and ancestors, or between developed and lesser-developed countries, or between religions or races. Influenced by the grief, losses, and despair that result from a world struggling to continue to survive, some women have reached out to reconnect with family members and old friends. Some women have gravitated to new relationships in unfamiliar places. All are seeking ways to comfort and soothe the collective pain.

Gotcha Covered: A Legacy of Service and Protection

The apron has existed as an object of practical design and as a signifier of social standing for both men and women for centuries. Previous generations of women signaled their status and roles through the shape, fabric, and style of their aprons, but it was not until after the mid-twentieth century that women in the western world attached feelings, initially of power and then of disempowerment, to the wearing of aprons.

During the 1930s and 1940s, many women in lower socio-economic groups had, through necessity, worked outside their homes, juggling family and job responsibilities, but it was uncommon for middle- and upper-class women to work outside the home. Despite this stay-at-home tradition, these middle/upper-class women had proudly gone to work during wartime, wearing headscarves and wielding hammers and blowtorches in service to their country. When the men returned to reclaim those jobs, the women returned to their homes. A systematic campaign to romanticize aprons as signifiers of domestic empowerment was carried out after the war to encourage these women to wear a variety of both utilitarian and fashion aprons. These aprons signified to postwar women, their families, and their guests the women's ownership of their kitchens, dining rooms, and parlors, in ways that are hard for many modern women to understand. When a woman of this era donned her apron, she was taken seriously. She felt important—the owner of her domain. The heyday of domestic aprons peaked in the late 1960s.

Not all women agreed with this view of womanhood. A recent article explains, "Women were either wearing aprons or reading briefs; the two identities seemed at war with another." (Hymowitz, 2008) Some women saw apron-wearing in the home as symbolic of servitude and disempowerment, and they advocated for women's liberation. They identified aprons and brassieres, among other items of clothing, as encumbrances on female advancement. By the 1970s, aprons had become symbolic of domestic servitude for many women, and liberated women discarded them and eventually disdained them. Except for utility or barbecue aprons, most women through the 1980s and early 1990s rarely ever wore aprons.

In the late 1990s and onward, some women developed newfound relationships with aprons. Today, there are apron exhibits in museums and in small and large communities worldwide. Vintage aprons sell on eBay, and women's magazines run stories on apron nostalgia and have sections devoted to apron crafts. Aprons have resurfaced as fashion accessories. *Anthropologie,* a high-end women's clothing and accessories chain, sells retro-inspired aprons in their stores across the nation. Ultra-high-fashion model Elizabeth Scokin sells her aprons for over $300 in tony stores in San Francisco and on the Internet. ("Haute Hostess Aprons by Elizabeth Scokin") Writing in the *Wall Street Journal,* Melanie Trottman noted that today's aprons "hug the body to show off curves, with colorful vampy designs that have little to do with sweating over a hot stove." (Trottman, 2005)

In the 2008 presidential election, issues of feminism and aprons surfaced, relative to both vice-presidential candidate Sarah Palin and presidential-primary candidate Hillary Clinton. Some Palin supporters noted that she tied on apron strings with pride, thus integrating feminism with femininity, while they accused Clinton of "hiding behind the apron strings." (Mia, ecomama.blogspot.com) Kay S. Hymowitz (2008) comments that Palin, a product of third-wave feminism, represented red-state feminists who are supposedly comfortable both with their feminist and their feminine side, while Clinton, a product of second-wave feminism, represented blue-state feminists who allegedly are dismissive of their feminine side.

Florence Nightingale is widely credited as the founder of modern nursing, beginning with her pioneering work with soldiers in the Crimean War in the 1850s. This was a time when women, especially women of elite classes, were not expected to be reformers. However, Nightingale, a product of upper-class England, became a champion reformer, single-handedly transforming the chaotic situation endured by the battlefield soldier into one with order and sanitation. To do this, she had to fight gender-based tyranny, both from within her own family and from the mostly male medical and military establishment within which she worked. Despite these social conditions, Nightingale was no champion of feminism. She believed that women should just get down to the business of doing what needed to be done and not complain that they were being held back by men. (Bostridge, 2008)

Nursing and aprons have been linked since the Middle Ages, when nuns who were attending the sick were depicted wearing aprons to protect their clothes. The nurse's costume of the late 1800s was similar to that worn by Victorian-era housemaids and nannies and, to some extent, that worn by religious sisters. However, the nurse's apron was designed not so much to fit in with other service identities, but rather as a matter of practicality to cover as much as possible the area likely to receive splatters from a nurse's work. Nightingale was a stickler for cleanliness, a notion almost unknown among medical providers of her day, and an apron could be easily changed when it was soiled.

Following the path established by Nightingale, nurses and nursing students in England, Australia, Canada, and the United States wore aprons, usually voluminous white ones that completely covered their dresses. This tradition continued until the late 1960s, both to protect the nurse and the patient and to signify to the public the powerful role of the nurse.

In the late 1960s, into the 1970s, many middle-class women, especially those who were nurses, bought into the myth of Superwoman. Nurses believed they could establish professional careers outside the home, while concurrently taking care of their families in the same way as women who stayed at home. Nurses who followed this path began to experience the same stresses as women who had always worked outside their homes. It was bittersweet; while nurses experienced enlightenment about the possibilities for their own personal and professional empowerment, they were often caught in the conflict of choosing between career and family. In the 1980s, some of these nurses opted out of the profession, while others stayed in, adjusting in one way or another to both professional and societal upheavals.

Nursing education responded to some of the second-wave feminist changes and moved away from apprentice-based training in hospitals towards education in colleges and universities. Concurrently, most student and professional nursing uniforms evolved away from aprons. Today nurses usually wear scrubs or lab coats, but aprons, either those made of lead or plastic, remain part of the required dress for nurses in some environments.

In the last part of the twentieth century, nurses became more autonomous, sometimes owning their own clinics and achieving positions of parity with some physicians. Ironically, during this same time, nurses became the most frequently targeted group of professional women to be exploited as sex symbols by the advertising and pornography industries. In almost all of these depictions, the "naughty nurse" is shown wearing an abbreviated form of an apron and sometimes not wearing much more than that, a fact not lost on organized nursing associations who have regularly, often successfully, lobbied against such depictions.

Quite unintentionally on my part, several of the foregoing historical details converged and led to this book. I am a registered nurse, educated in a university in the 1960s, after most nurses had ceased wearing aprons as part of their uniform. I spent my early adult years personally and professionally struggling for gender parity. Aprons, correctly or not, were one of the symbols my generation perceived as emblematic of servitude for women, and we rejected such talismans, both as part of our nursing uniforms and in our kitchens.

The aprons in this anthology derive from a collection of mid-twentieth-century vintage aprons saved from the households of two sisters—my aunt and my mother. Both women were excellent cooks and full-time homemakers who wore aprons for everyday and for special occasions all their adult lives. My mother was widowed young and subsequently moved a number of times before her final move into a nursing home. Along the way, all her possessions, aprons among them, were discarded. After she died, only three of her most recent aprons—from what had surely at one time been almost a hundred aprons—remained in her goods. On the other hand, her sister, my Aunt Katherine, lived in the same house from her wedding day until the day, sixty years later, when she moved into a retirement apartment. Almost fifty of her aprons survived those years, and in 2006 I inherited the boxes that contained those aprons.

About a month later—forty years after our graduation—my nursing class held a reunion in my home. Surprising ourselves, we were drawn to the vintage aprons I had inherited and we resolved to create something—a story, a poem, a visual creation—inspired by them, and to use any proceeds that came from our endeavor to help fund the efforts of other nurses who needed help to provide health care services. From this beginning came The Nurses' Apron Partnership, our web site, and ultimately this book.

By mid-2007, fifty nurses had signed on to adopt an apron, contribute to the book, and support the vision. One early adopter ultimately had to drop out and her apron was readopted. One apron was accidentally adopted by two nurses. One nurse adopted two similar aprons as a pair. Eventually, one nurse in Kenya joined the group of American nurses, adopting an apron abandoned at the last moment by another nurse who had to withdraw, leaving forty-nine nurses in the final mix. The nurses were asked to respond to the adopted apron from their heart and soul—to let the apron speak to them, and to let their spirit hear and reply in some creative way. Some of the nurses responded from their theology, some from memory or history, some from resistance or struggle to understand their journey, and some from a point of view of fantasy or playfulness. These creative contributions have been gathered into this anthology.

The contributors' ages range from twenty-something to mid-eighties. Their nursing educations range from hospital-diploma schools to associate, baccalaureate, and master's degrees to doctoral preparation. The oldest nurse-participant was born soon after women in the United States achieved the right to vote. She graduated from nursing school in 1945, just at the end of World War II.

The majority of the contributors are nurses born in the late 1930s and the 1940s. They came of age in the 1950s and 1960s during the second wave of feminism. The younger nurses who contributed to this anthology were born in the late 1960s, the 1970s, and the early 1980s. They came of age in the 1990s and were influenced by the third wave of feminism. All of the contributors have been influenced by fourth-wave feminism.

Several broad categories emerged from the submissions, reflecting differing aspects of the creator's spirit. These categories are arranged in four sections: *Aprons as Symbols of Healing*, *Aprons as Symbols of Identity and Service*, *Aprons as Symbols of Comfort*, and *Aprons as Symbols of Imagination and Creativity*.

Some of the stories are works of art fashioned by skilled artisans. Some submissions are more works of love (or maybe not!), like the aprons many of us made in home economics class in eighth grade. Some contributors wrote thousands of words, and some struggled to complete a paragraph. One contributor said that even if she never saw her written piece in print, the process of doing it had allowed a part of herself that had gaped inside to heal.

How can a humble apron have such power?

These aprons speak a language that binds women to one another in a way that seems to be universally recognized. They are reflective of women—especially of women who are nurses—as wise healers and nurturers. These are conversations written from a female view, in a female voice, about rituals transmitted from ancestors to descendants.

The stories are evocative. They inform us of our past and provide guidance for our future. They allow us to go back, to reconnect, to complete, and to gather energy for going forward.

This apron anthology should be read sitting in a special place, maybe with a cup of coffee or tea in hand, perhaps with a mother or daughter or best friend nearby. The stories are conversations. They beg to be shared. Sometimes the stories are simple and homespun; sometimes they are extraordinarily poignant and complex. Ultimately, this is a book about the wisdom of a simple garment that historically has been seen as both empowering and disempowering—that covers and protects—that signifies nurturing and healing—*Gotcha Covered!*

Ginger T. Manley
June 2009

Part One: *Aprons as Symbols of Healing*

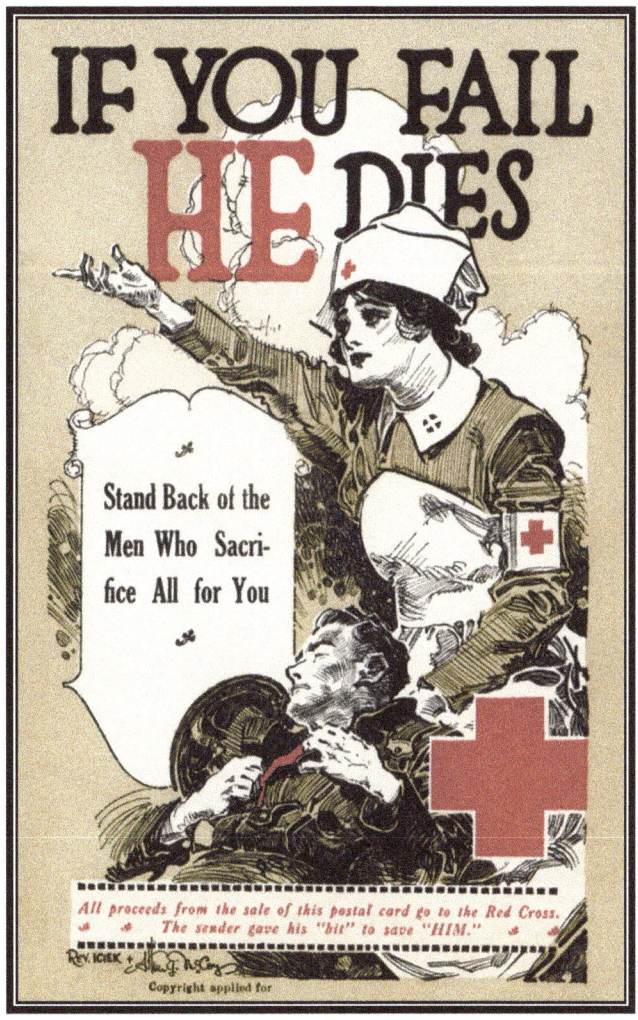

© Zwerdling Nursing Archives, used with permission.

Aprons As Symbols of Healing

Ginger T. Manley

Nursing involves more than the skills of nursing. It is about identity and shared myths and shared memories, which nurses construct with other nurses.

Susan Gelfand Malka, *Daring to Care*

Until the late nineteenth century, the sick were usually cared for in the home by family members. During the Middle Ages, care of the sick began to take place in convents or abbeys, where the caregivers were members of a religious order. Both medieval housewives and nuns wore aprons while attending the ill, not as symbols of their healing role or for sanitation, but because aprons were a part of female clothing of that time.

Florence Nightingale's experiences in the Crimean War in 1854 set the stage for the formal preparation and training of nurses as we know the profession today. Nightingale trained as a nurse at the Institute of Deaconesses in Kaiserwerth, Germany, and afterwards volunteered to serve in Crimea. She was horrified by the chaos she encountered there, and in reaction to these conditions, developed her authoritarian positions about the necessity for cleanliness and discipline among nurses. In 1860 she began the Nightingale Training School for Nurses in London—the first organized program in the world that taught the basics of modern nursing care.

In the late 1800s, the idealized Victorian view of upper-class women elevated the female above the rest of earth's creatures. As the Nightingale model of nursing developed, it paralleled this Victorian view, creating the standard of a nurse who was both proper and pious, only a small step removed from a nun. For most of the next century, the Nightingale model would be the standard for hospital-based nursing education worldwide.

In the Nightingale model, nursing students, who were almost always women, lived together in a building adjacent to a hospital. These students worked long hours, usually learning as apprentices as they worked. Nightingale designed the first nursing uniform—a full-length dress with long sleeves and a high neck, which was covered by a full apron that wrapped around to the back of the dress. Usually the apron was stiffly starched, both for fashion and for protection. One account from early twentieth-century wartime urges nurses to keep their aprons well-starched to keep the body lice of patients from crawling to the nurse. ("Why do QA Army nurses wear grey dresses and berets?" Q & A Forum)

Almost every subsequent hospital nursing school adopted a version of this uniform for both its students and graduates. By many accounts, student nurses who wore the early aprons felt great affection for them. The positive experience of tying their apron around their waist signified a transformation from a *nobody* to a *somebody*. According to an account from the U.S. Naval Research Center:

> *During World War I in the operating room and in dressing work in the hospital wards, the War Nurse wore this white utility apron. It was a most unromantic apron, adopted to simplify the ever-present French laundry problem, but it was a badge of service coveted by thousands of untrained women.*
> ("Nurses and the U.S. Navy. 1917–1919—Red Cross and Army nurses' uniforms.")

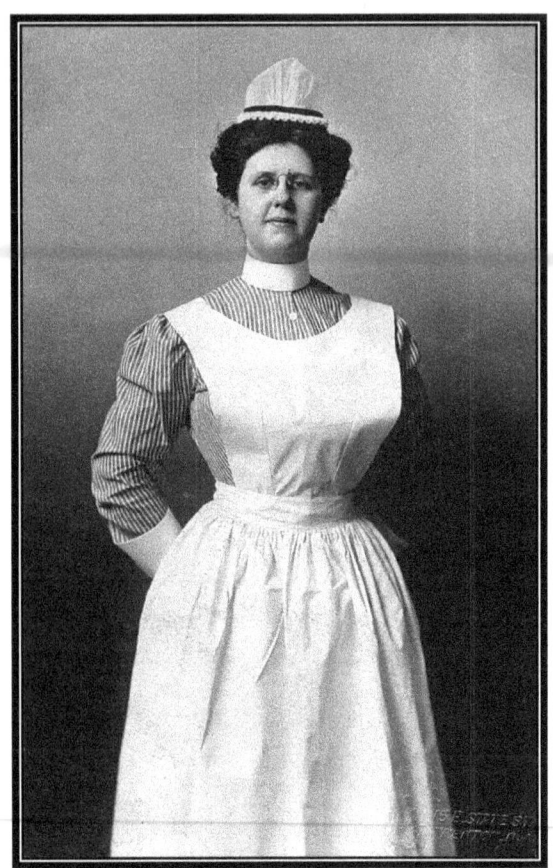

1890s era nurse in full wrap apron.
© Zwerdling Nursing Archives, used with permission.

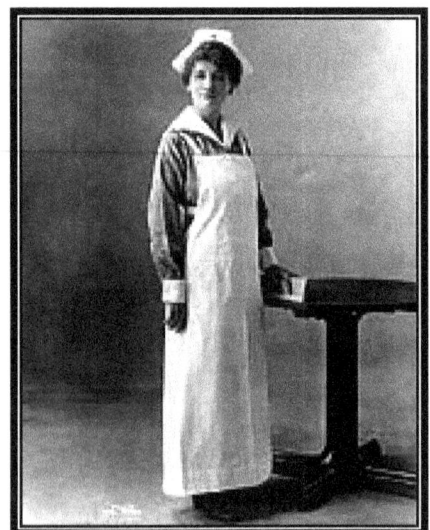

War Nurse Uniform c. 1916,
"Nurses and the U.S. Navy. 1917–1919
—Red Cross and Army nurses' uniforms"

In the early twentieth century, as hospital training programs merged into university settings, the uniform with an apron migrated with many of them, and eventually bib-front aprons replaced the full, wrap-around aprons. By the mid-twentieth century, clothing styles had evolved into shorter and less voluminous outfits, and nursing fashion changed accordingly. When washable fabrics became more available, aprons were modified again. By the late 1960s, many nursing programs, both hospital-based and university-based, had done away with aprons.

Many nursing schools now have web sites that display the evolution of aprons worn by their students. Several schools have permanent displays of dolls dressed in the student uniforms of each era. Some programs kept a simplified version of the apron as more of a fashion touch than for its function, until the middle 1980s when scrubs and lab coats began to provide coverage and identification for the wearer. If nurses needed to wear aprons in contaminated environments, such aprons were made of plastic or disposable paper.

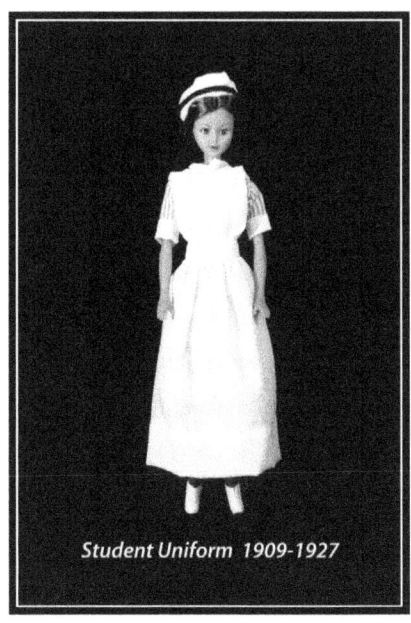
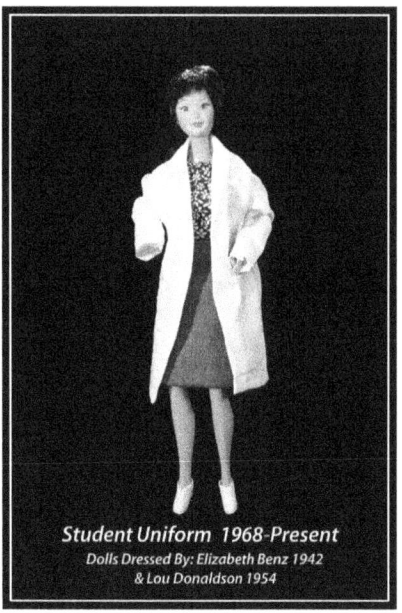

Images of the earliest and most recent student uniforms of Vanderbilt University School of Nursing.
© 2008, Vanderbilt University School of Nursing, used with permission.

Nurses' aprons were the original impetus for Avis Smith's master's research, done in Australia in the late 1990s. Years earlier, while working as chief pharmacist with the Royal Flying Doctor Service, she traveled to remote Australian communities. "It was during such visits that I noticed the difference to the persona of a woman as soon as she put on her starched white apron and (in those days) her starched white veil." (Avis Smith, e-mail to Ginger Manley, March 6, 2008) Smith devoted a full chapter of her thesis to the study of nurses' aprons. She concludes, "The white apron as the outer layer of the nurse's clothes-body complex has, within public perception, become firmly associated with professional (feminine) care and comfort. . . . The white apron of nursing has always exerted a powerful psychological as well as visual effect." (Smith, 2003, p.64) Projecting forward, Smith wonders, "If nurses are visually defined by what they wear but there is no common fashion component such as the white apron in the forthcoming twenty-first century, will professional integrity be automatically assumed for them if they 'dress like the people'?" (Smith, 2003, p. 67)

In his award-winning book, *Postcards of Nursing: A Worldwide Tribute* (2004), Michael Zwerdling, a registered nurse, published hundreds of his vast collection of vintage postcards showing nurse images. These images "include comic and stereotypical images . . . and show the progression of the apron representing service to humanity to service in the name of a commercial product presented by a maid . . ." (Michael Zwerdling, e-mail to Ginger Manley, April 12, 2008) Additionally, the book contains many photographs of royalty and actresses costumed as nurses, almost all wearing an apron.

Susan Gelfand Malka (2007) defines the progression of nursing culture and nursing education in the United States as eras defined by aprons. Malka compares and contrasts nursing's journey as it parallels feminism, noting that from both lanes of this socio-cultural road there was, at the same time, both sympathy and disdain for the other side.

A compelling new book, *Nurse: A World of Care* (Jaret, 2008), includes full-page photos of contemporary nurses at work the world over, wearing scrubs, student uniforms, everyday clothes, saris, religious habits, black aprons, lab coats, shorts and tank tops, hazmat suits, jeans, Muslim headscarves, and traditional white aprons and caps. The text and the photos confirm how powerful the presence of a nurse can be, giving "voice not through words but through actions" (p. 37), no matter what clothing that nurse is wearing.

In this section, the voices of several nurses speak of their connection—or not—to aprons, and especially to the personal identity of being a nurse. Aprons historically have symbolized nurturing and healing, and their powerful legacy continues to influence nurses and the public today.

In Our Voices:
The Legacy of Nursing

GOTCHA COVERED: A LEGACY OF SERVICE AND PROTECTION

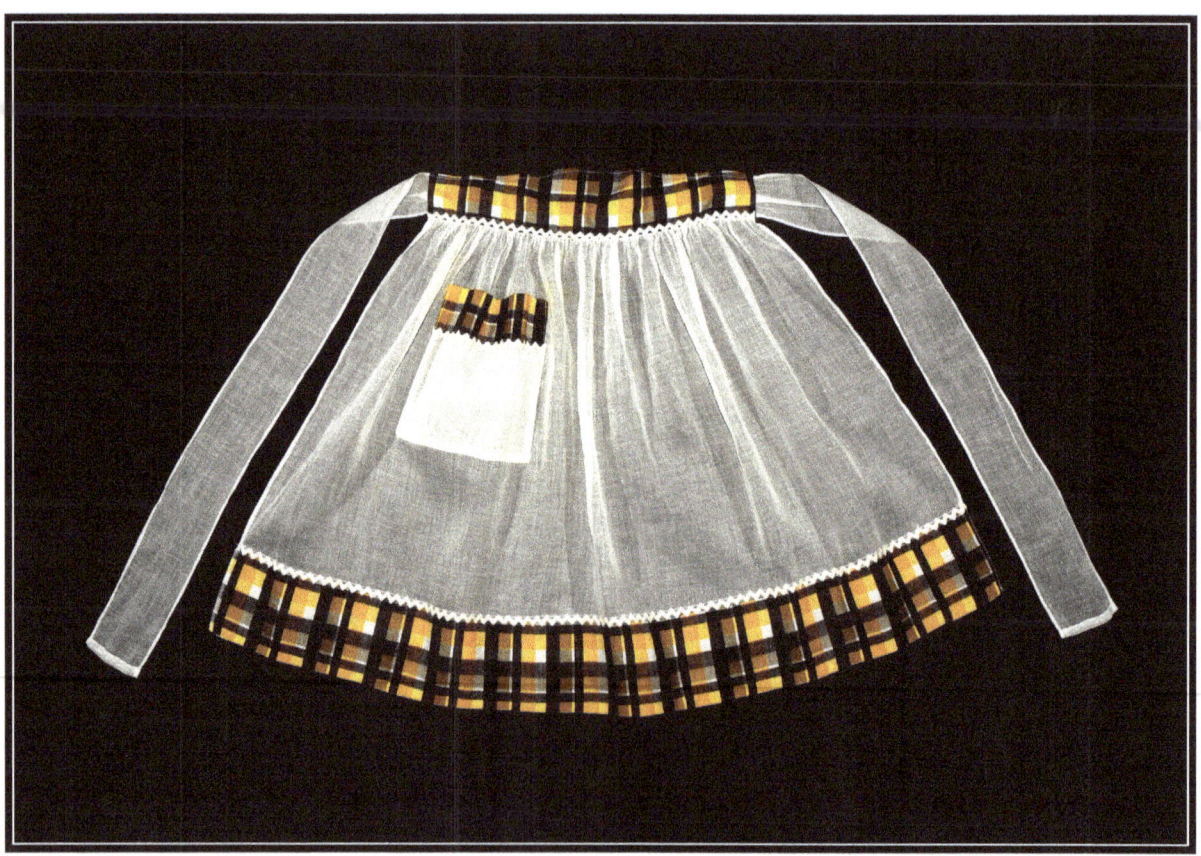

Adopted August 8, 2007 by Kathleen L. Wolff

Kathleen L. Wolff

This unwrinkled apron, adorned with orderly geometric shapes, represents what I am not. No plaids or stiff-starched fabric for me. I flee from too much structure and orderliness, staying just a hair's breadth from chaos most of the time. Having balanced single motherhood and full-time nurse-practitionering for many years, my mothering, cooking, and housekeeping bore little resemblance to those of one who would wear this apron. There was little need for a cooking apron in my kitchen—and a lab coat, not an apron, symbolized my role as a nurse.

This apron is what I am not. And I wonder, how might my life be different had I been more like this apron?

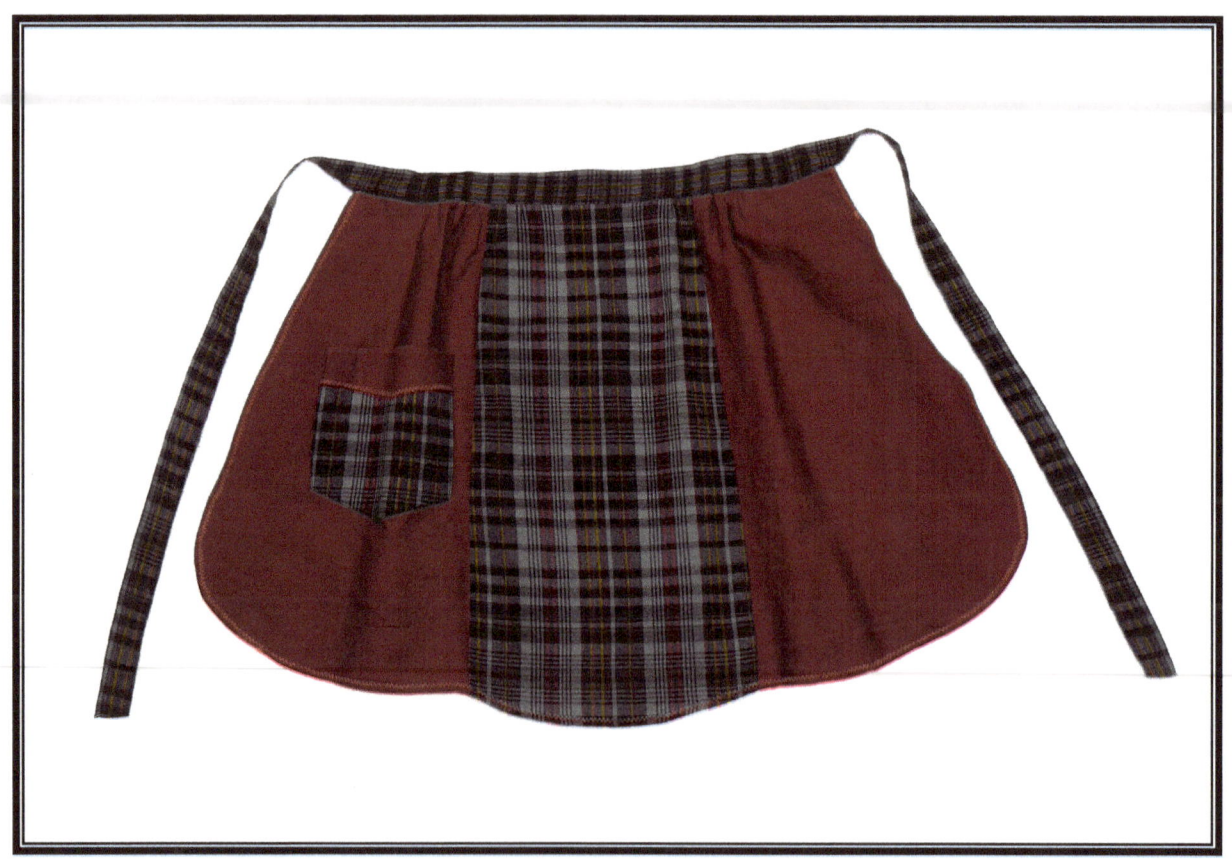

Adopted March 28, 2007 by Marilyn Bache Sonnenberg

Marilyn Bache Sonnenberg

As a youngster, I visited aunts and uncles working at resorts and, with them, helped prepare the dining rooms for the arrival of the guests. I can still remember my uncle, a headwaiter, returning to his room to steam-press his "whites" so that the creases in his pants would be crisp when he returned to the dining room for the next meal. Watching and listening to family conversations, I learned very early that knowing the preferences of guests and providing special attention would result in rewards, both in the sense of great feelings of accomplishment, as well as in great tips. I could not wait to be old enough to actually work as a waitress myself.

Eventually, I too had a station in dining rooms alongside older members of my family. Every summer and Christmas holiday, through the time I received my master's degree, I worked as a waitress in resort hotels. In my memory, these were halcyon times.

I met other college students and immigrants who were getting started in the United States, just as my family had. We all lived in cabins or dormitory rooms, were part of a special society that played when others worked, and worked when others were on holidays or vacations. And we had fun. In my memory, these were times of full immersion in life. Then too, by donning my apron alongside others, I was able to earn enough money to cover college expenses during the academic year. My income then was greater than I was able to earn later as a new BSN graduate.

It has now been a long time since I have worn an apron—any apron. As a nurse, and as a faculty member of a nursing college, I worked intentionally to remove vestiges of servanthood from my attire. However, when I look back on experiences that shaped my self-image, values, ambition, and work ethic, this little apron is a powerful symbol of who I was, and who I am today.

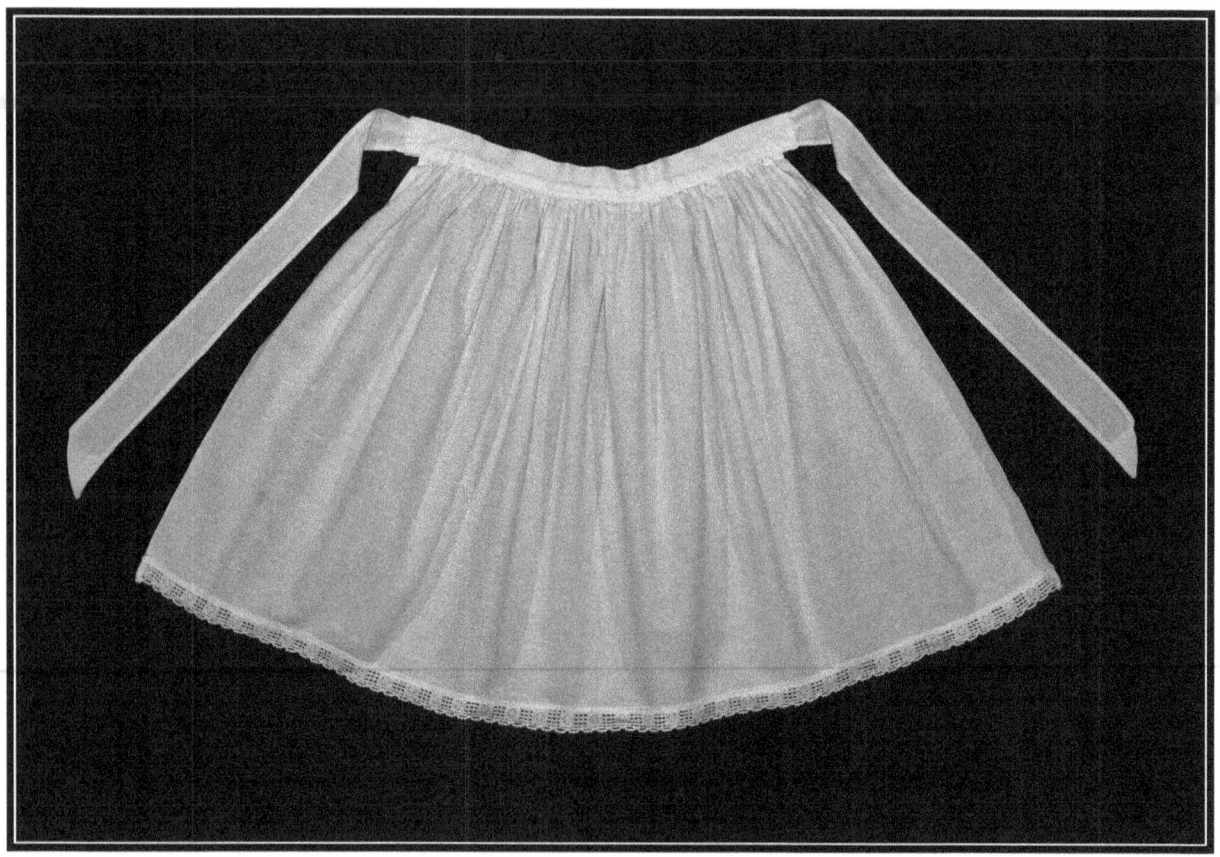

Adopted March 8, 2007 by Karen L. Starr

Karen L. Starr

Touching the fabric of the crisp, white, organdy, adopted apron, trimmed in several rows of crochet work, almost instantly transported me back to the object of my adulation as a young girl—Cherry Ames. Cherry was my heroine when I was ten years old. When the authors, Helen Wells and Julie Tatham, portrayed Cherry's adventures in nursing, I fantasized being her and doing what she did. From Cherry's days as a student nurse to her active-duty stint in the Army Nurse Corps, she was my role model for what a nurse should be.

I held onto the dream of being a nurse after I had given up the idea of being a movie star. To a ten-year-old, these two professions seemed to be so much alike. Both were glamorous, larger-than-life, challenging, and filled with drama. The former, however, seemed more attainable. Life experiences delayed my dreams of becoming a registered nurse. The first hurdle was erected when my mother told me that I could never be a nurse because she said that I couldn't stand the sight of blood. The second hurdle was one I put up myself when I came to believe *I'm not smart enough*.

I graduated in 1976 at the age of thirty-two with my baccalaureate degree in nursing from the University of Missouri. I was incredulous. I had achieved my lifelong goal! When I finally began to work in the field of nursing, I had to pinch myself to believe I was actually doing what had once been only a plan and a dream.

The larger-than-life, dramatic, and glamorous aspects of nursing faded within a few months. The challenge of doing something I love has never faded.

I even managed to become that Army nurse that Cherry Ames so aptly role-modeled for me. I was commissioned in the Army Nurse Corps on September 23, 1977, and spent four years on active duty, and twenty-four years in the active reserve. I retired in 2005, after twenty-eight years of service.

I cannot imagine doing anything else. Nursing has become a part of who I am, maybe who I always was. I will be working for as long as my legs will hold me up and my mind is alert to the challenge of the tasks at hand.

Gotcha Covered: A Legacy of Service and Protection

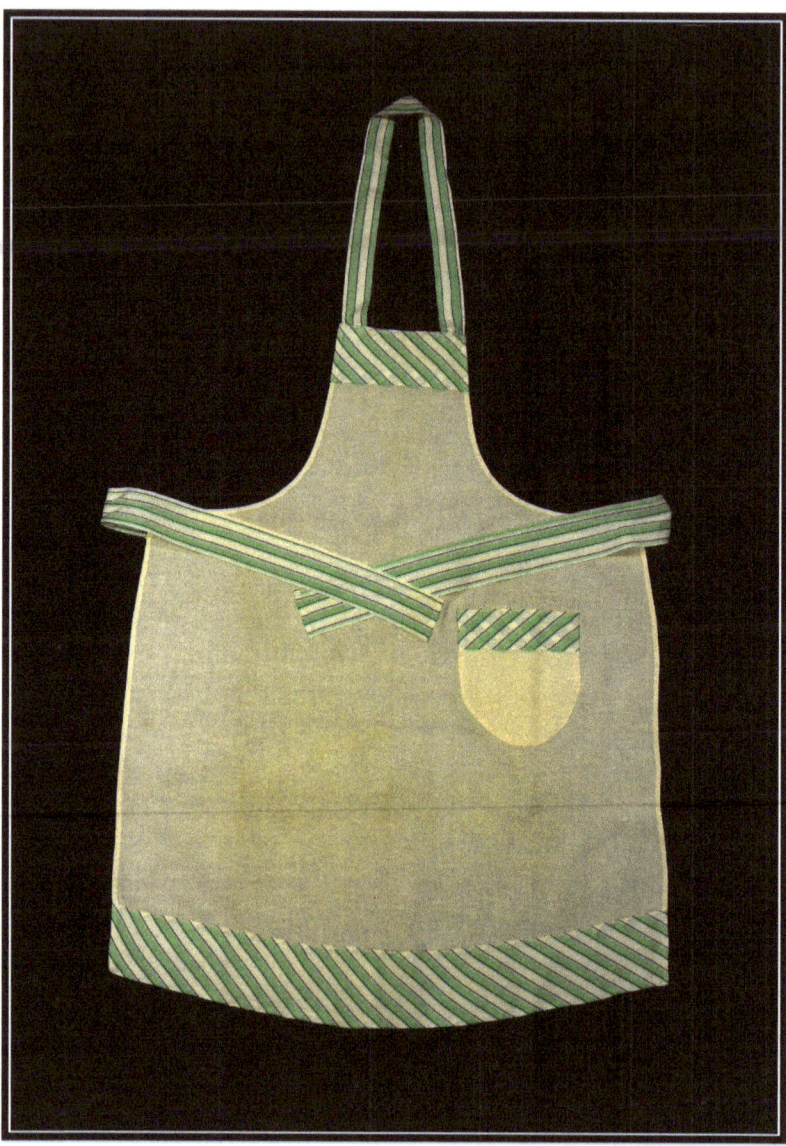

Adopted March 11, 2007 by Joan Crosland Chapman Sughrue

Joan Crosland Chapman Sughrue

To my dearest adopted apron,

When I first saw your photograph, I thought, "How can I not adopt this one? It looks just like me! I'm an apron person after all."

Your white front is trimmed in the traditional fashion of the candy striper—long known for its association with nursing. The green stripes reminded me of my start in nursing through the Girl Scout program in which I worked for a badge as hospital aide. At the young age of fourteen, I knew I had found my vocation, my calling—my passion.

Adoption is a very personal decision. It should never be taken lightly as the responsibilities are enormous . . . but the rewards are great. I welcome you into my sisterhood of family, friends, and colleagues.

When I was in nursing school, my family adopted a little girl, Barbara Lynn. She fulfilled the dreams of my mother and stepfather who had lost their baby girl, Cheryl, after a few short weeks of life. Lynn has a purity of spirit that shines in her heart and in her deeds. What a blessing this sister has been to our family.

My biological sisters, Judy and Ginger, have steadfastly been my friends as we grew into adulthood. No matter our quarrels, we know we can count on each other in times of joy and in times of sorrow. The best part of our relationship is that I get to be the know-it-all, for you see, I am the nurse.

Some of my best friends are also my sisters in nursing. Pat was my first friend after I moved away to work in my newly adopted hometown of Charleston, SC. We met during orientation at the hospital where we were employed. Our friendship is now thirty-five years plus and still going strong.

My friend, Lynne, joined the nursing sisterhood after enjoying two other careers as a teacher and business owner. I was an inspiration for her—or so she says. Our friendship is now twenty-five years plus and still going strong. Pat and Lynne have also become my adopted sisters through the love and support that has endured throughout the years.

My colleagues in nursing are also special sisters (and brothers). Relationships change when you identify as a nurse. The bonds of shared experiences unite us. We are unique, each in our own way, as nursing provides diverse pathways to help others. We can hold one another in regard even when our practices and viewpoints are different.

Therefore, my dearest adopted apron, I welcome you into my sisterhood with the most wonderful women I know. You are the symbol of my passion for nursing—pure and elegantly trimmed. You cradle my hopes for the future and your ties gently bind me with my nursing sisters. The responsibilities of being a nurse have been enormous . . . but the rewards have been even greater.

Welcome to my sisterhood, my family.

GOTCHA COVERED: A LEGACY OF SERVICE AND PROTECTION

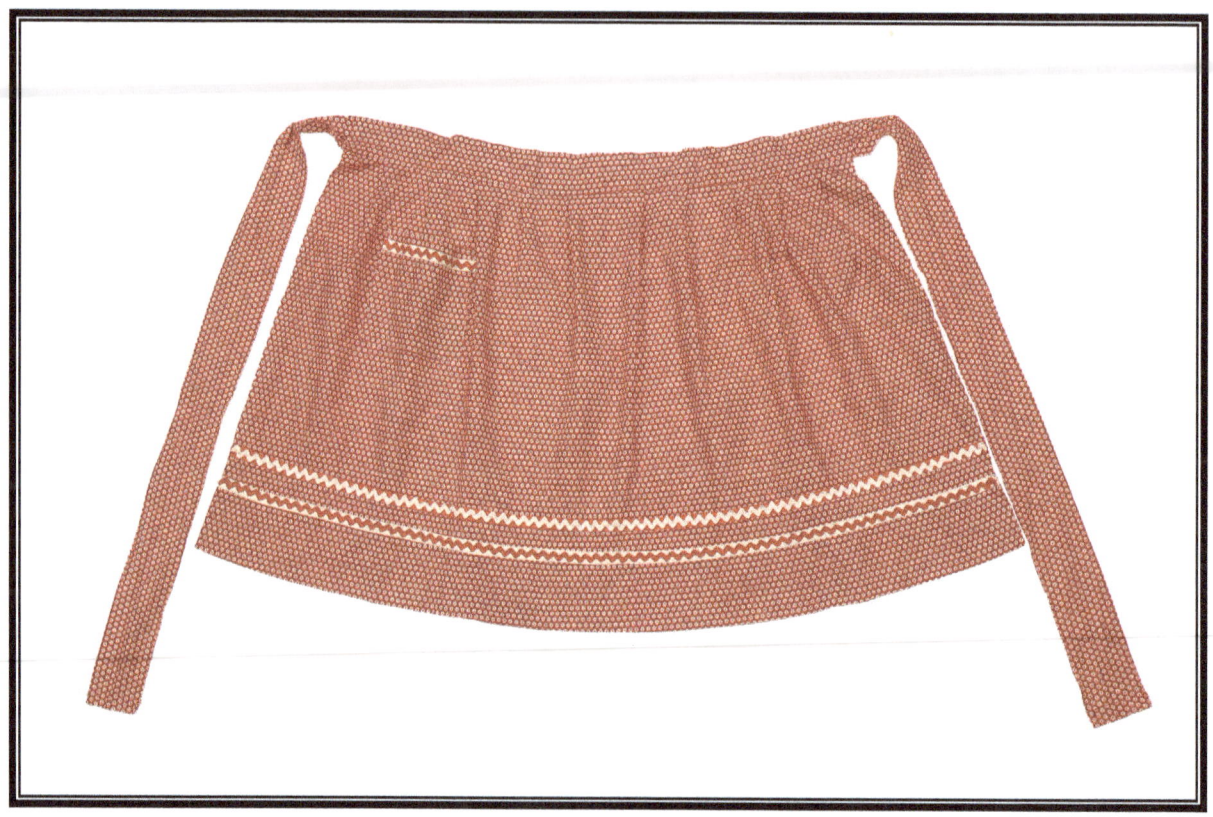

Adopted March 17, 2007 by Mary Jo Reimer

Mary Jo Reimer

Life through the early 1960s was very different from what we women experience now. As I was growing up, I had a strong interest in the healthcare world, but my ambition waned as I allowed myself to become indoctrinated in the prevailing idea that a woman's place is in the home raising children. Both my mother and my older sister had large families, and had little time for wearing fancy aprons, but they were very happy and content with their lives.

With such role models, little did I dream I would be working outside the home throughout my life. Indeed, I became the consummate career woman. I never even owned an apron. I preferred smart suits and trashy shoes—colorful high heels with bows, ankle straps, and open toes.

Although I spent many years in the accounting field and experienced a pleasant level of success, I was never really content—but I made do. My restlessness propelled me to change jobs frequently, but always to a higher rung up the ladder. During this time, I was married and raising children. Everyone thought I had it all. Along the way, I became controller of a pension plan located in Los Angeles. While I was there, I hired Pat, a young man who became my good friend.

Unfortunately, in the early 1980s, my life was torn apart by a heartbreaking divorce. Pat was a source of great comfort to me, not only as a top-notch employee, but as a caring and reliable friend.

As I am sure we all recall, that same period of time also ushered in the advent of the AIDS epidemic. Pat contracted the disease and suffered a painful course until his death some two years later. As he deteriorated, he had no one to help him through his ordeal. His family was a distance away from him, not only geographically, but emotionally as well. It was natural that I should help him and I was glad to do so.

It was rewarding to make a difference in someone's life, although we who cared also needed support and counseling as we supported our buddy. For a diversion from such overwhelming sadness, I did stand-up comedy. My persona was a glamorous and flamboyant mother. I wore my hair spiked, tight-fitting dresses with short skirts, and knee-high, red leather boots with very high heels. Again, it was a far cry from housewifely aprons and genteel afternoon teas. I was with APLA (AIDS Project Los Angeles) for six years and was honored to be the recipient of their award for volunteer of the year in 1990.

By this time, my children were all living independently, and I was in a position to quit working and enroll in school. My interest in the healthcare world had never completely disappeared, and after a couple of classes just for fun I decided to become a nurse. It felt right. For four years, year-round, I studied hard, engrossed in my classes and clinicals, and enjoyed every minute of them. I also switched to wearing plain white shoes—without high heels.

At the age of sixty, I became a registered nurse with an associate degree. The day of my RN boards was one of the happiest days of my life—and also, a great relief. My goal was to work in an AIDS hospice, and upon graduation that is exactly what I did. In the year 2001, I joined the Peace Corps and was sent to South Africa to continue in the battle against AIDS.

I am now in my seventies, and I continue to work because I find what I do to be so rewarding. Being an RN has not only fed me literally, but spiritually as well. Thank goodness the "pink ghetto" days attributed to nursing are long gone. Society has come to realize what an important role we play in life—and in death.

No one told me it would be an easy career, but it has been worth every minute I have put into it. The apron I have adopted is one that is colorful, but otherwise plain and sturdy—a metaphor for my life as a nurse.

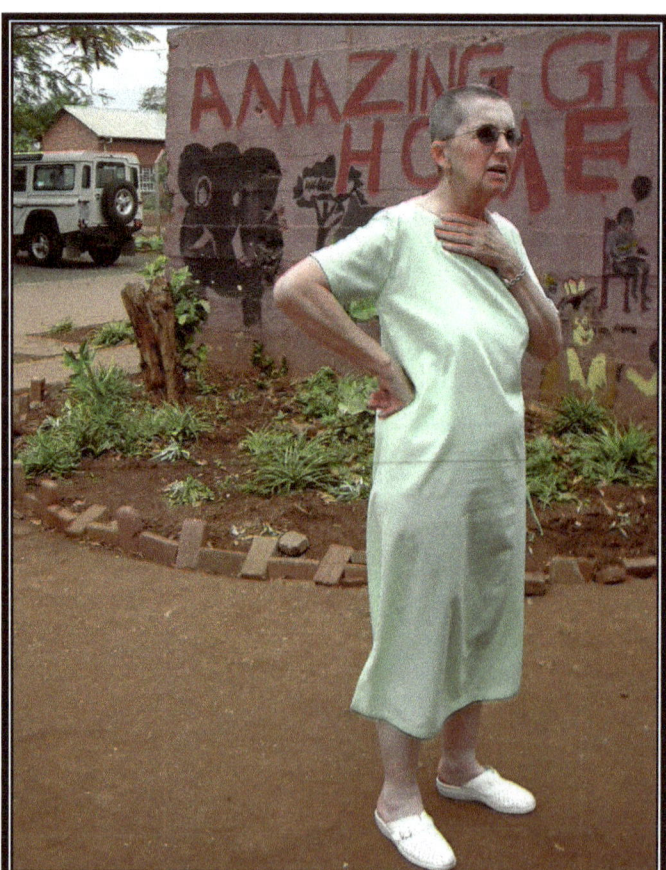

Mary Jo Reimer spent two years in Melanane, South Africa, in the Peace Corps, where she worked at Peace Haven, a home for orphaned children, some with HIV/AIDS. She was addressed there as "gogo," or grandmother, a sign of respect for this then 60-something year-old RN. Photo by Nicole Itano, used with permission.

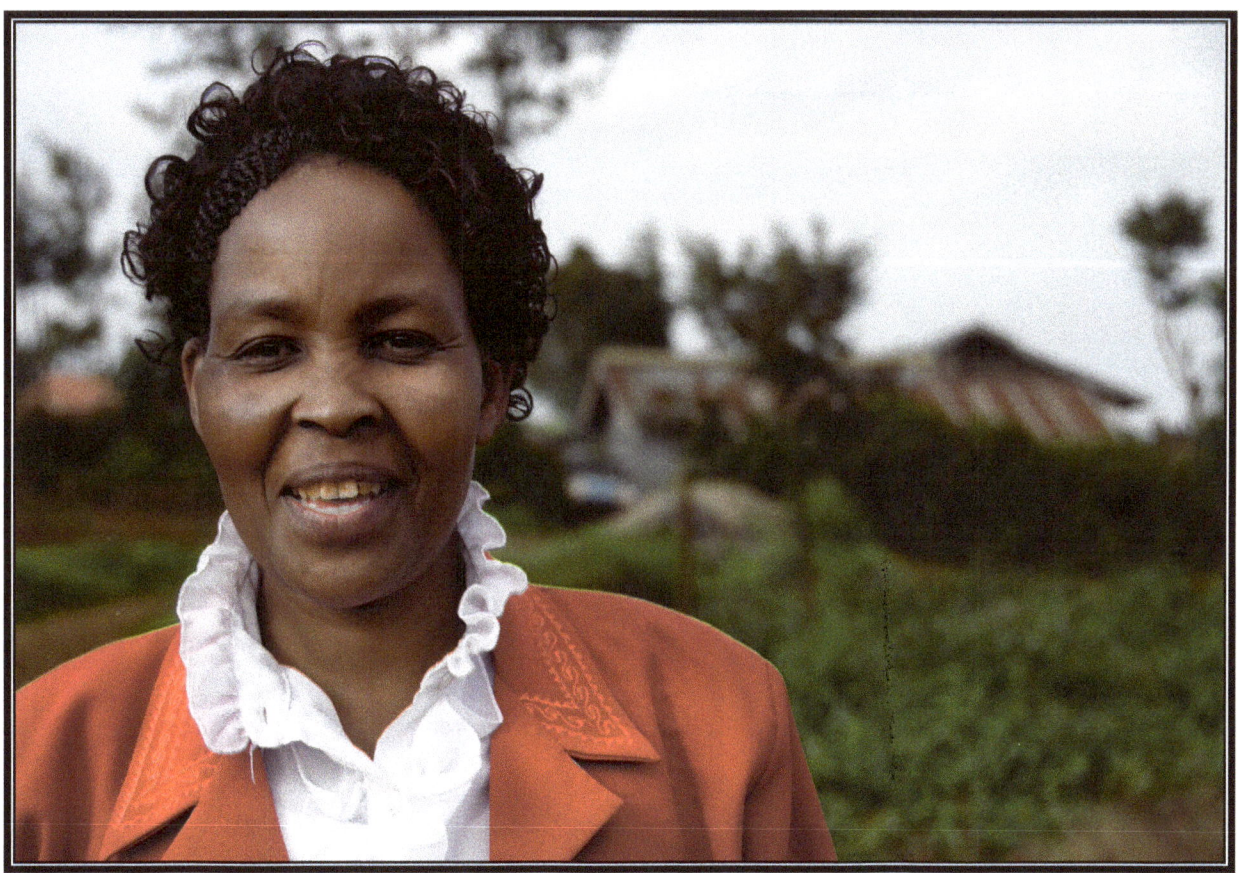

Jocelyn Macharia R.N. lives in Central Kenya where she owns her own clinic providing primary and maternity care. She is the first Kenyan nurse to receive a micro-credit loan from Burning Bush, Inc., partnered with donors from The Nurses' Apron Partnership, for her graduate studies in Community Pastoral Care and HIV/AIDS at St. Paul's University in Limuru, Kenya. Photo by Stacey Irvin.

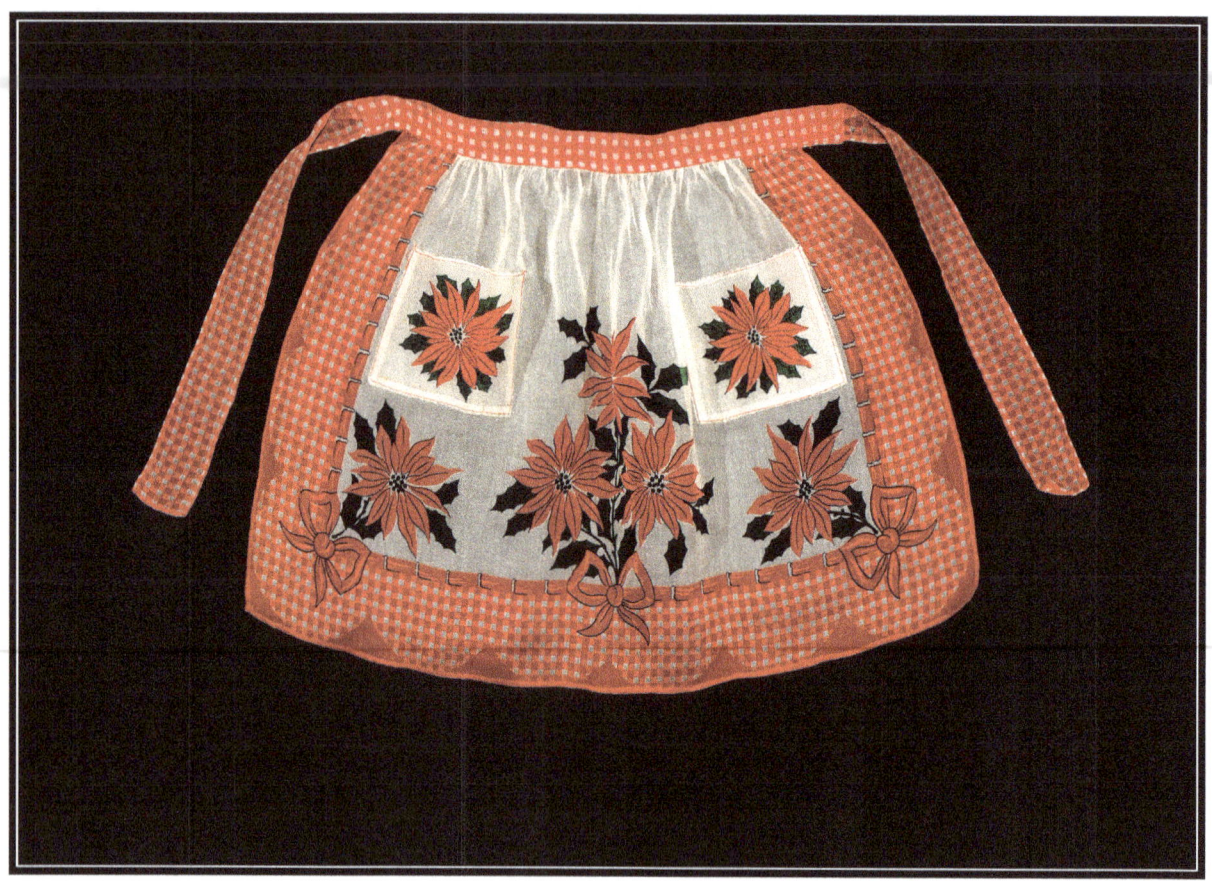

Adopted November 10, 2006 by Barbara Siddens Vinson

Barbara Siddens Vinson

I am one of four children born during World War II, while my dad was serving in the Navy. In 1951, when I was eight years old, I contracted polio in the epidemic. I had a curvature of the spine with muscular atrophy and was in bed for one year. I was home-schooled, and I wore a corset-type brace until I was a sophomore in high school. I had to exercise and swim a lot, and am blessed to have no visible effects of that horrible disease. School was easy for me and I spent very little energy on my studies. Sometime in my junior year of high school, I decided to become a nurse. I was awarded a full academic scholarship to Vanderbilt School of Nursing and I graduated in 1966 with a BSN.

I was married in 1968 and we had three daughters. I had to wear another corset-type brace for the second and third pregnancies, but I worked right up until the day they were born. I worked full-time as a nurse—and still do—and have loved my experiences and the patients I have served.

In the 1920s, my maternal grandparents started a tradition of family beach vacations, a ritual which my mother's sisters and their families continue today. I, too, have started a tradition. Our family makes and decorates Christmas cookies together. I have an apron that I have worn every year since 1973, when our girls were in the "Mother's Day Out" program. Through kindergarten and on to elementary school, we made Christmas cookies for them to share with their classmates and friends and neighbors. This cookie-making experience has become a tradition that is as much a part of Christmas as our sharing of gifts with each other. Now these same children come from Wisconsin, Texas, New York, Kentucky, and from all over Tennessee with their little ones to decorate Christmas cookies together. I watch my grandchildren with their own aprons, up to their elbows in flour and sugar, rolling out the dough, cutting out cookies, baking them, and then decorating them with colored icing and sprinkles, knowing they will share them with their little friends and neighbors.

It takes a lot of energy for me today to get all the things together—to clean and press my apron and the ones the little ones will wear, to make dough ahead of time, to plan the date, and then to keep things moving and organized. I try to step back and watch my children helping their own, sharing the joy of creating to give to others—and, of course, nibbling along the way. I love my life and the joys I have known, shared, and taught in some small way.

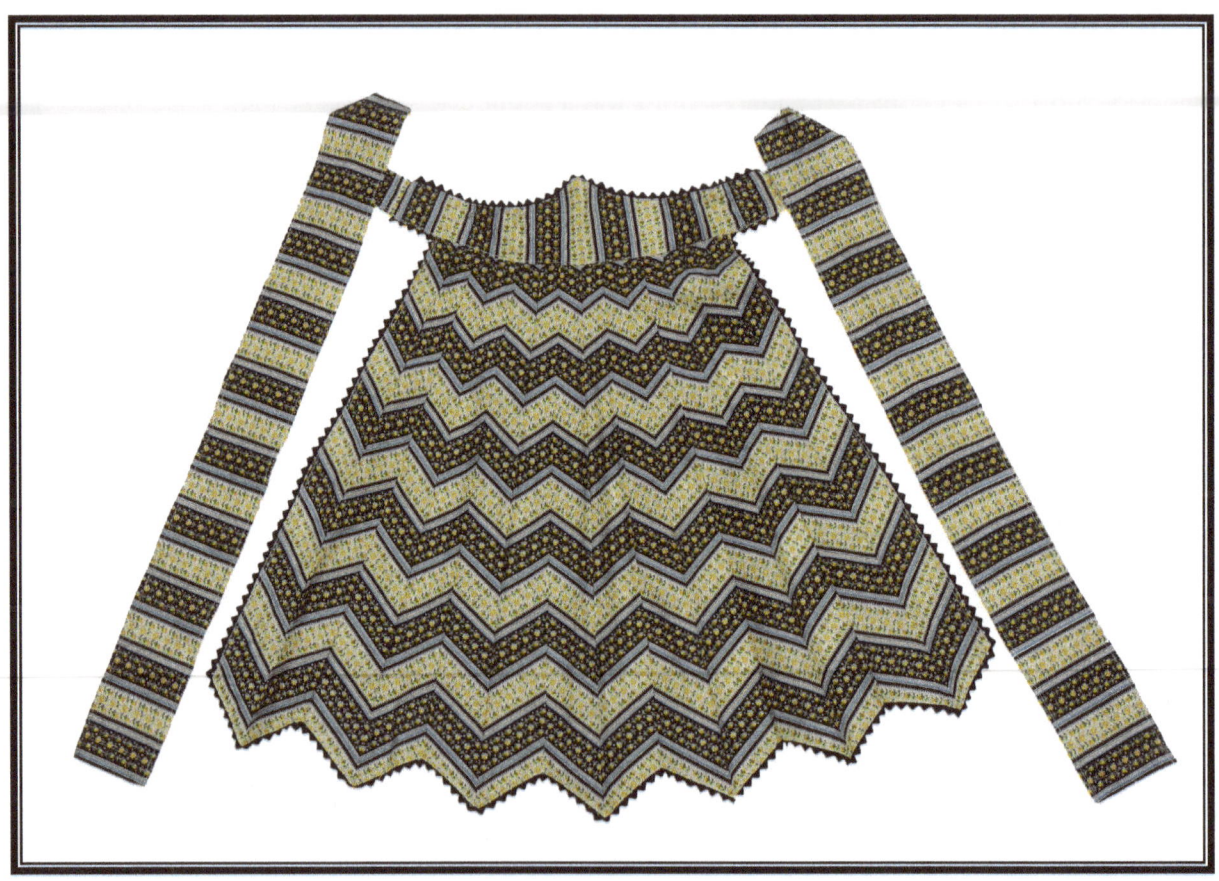

Adopted June 11, 2007 by Judith B. Collins

Judith B. Collins

As a late adopter, I received almost the last apron available. Despite this circumstance, the apron did speak to me. The fun pattern reminds me of the zigzags of life, and the straight lines on the apron strings seem to bring us back to our roots. The apron-tie symbolically ties us together throughout generations.

Looking back, aprons have had a wonderful place in my memory since I was a little girl. I had three strong women as influences in my life—maternal grandmother, mother, and maternal aunt. I clearly remember my grandmother wearing a full-coverage, vest-like apron she made for her many homemaker duties, as cook, master seamstress, gardener, canner, etc. One Christmas, I found my grandmother making doll clothes. She very cleverly told me that Mrs. Claus had asked her to be a helper. Surprise—one of the new doll dresses matched my grandmother's apron.

The memory of aprons ties to the next generation—my mother and aunt. Aprons were always a must while working in the kitchen. This was especially true for my mother who was a home economics teacher. The apron was her uniform for cooking, sewing, and housework. However, the protocol was she always removed her apron before sitting down at the dinner table. My maiden, schoolteacher aunt was very proper and always wore an apron in the kitchen. She traveled the world and used to bring colorful aprons back as souvenirs from many different countries.

Growing up, for special occasions and holidays there were fancy organza or theme aprons. I vividly remember the unique apron that had a plastic hoop frame that fit around the waist, and different holiday aprons could be slipped onto the frame in a gathered fashion. My favorites were Thanksgiving and Christmas.

Thanks to the Apron Project, I had the revelation that the apron-tie to my generation and profession was the white apron of my nursing uniform. Our University of North Carolina uniform was a navy-blue dress with a starched, detachable collar and cuffs, and the dress was covered by a starched white apron. The apron had pockets for the tools of our trade—bandage scissors, patient assignment notes, pens, drug cards, etc. How could I ever forget the white pearlized buttons that were removed before laundering and then reattached with metal pins through the loop on the back of the button, for the collar, cuffs, and apron? Boy could that make you late for clinicals unless you were organized.

When I became a homemaker, I continued the generational apron-ties, but only on special occasions. I used a pretty apron to protect my party outfit, but of course, according to my mother's protocol, I removed the apron before going to the table. There was a slight break in the apron-ties after I had a son. I never remember having him wear an apron, even baking cookies or dyeing Easter eggs. What a shame.

However, with the next generation—our grandchildren—the apron tradition was rebirthed with the annual cookie and cupcake bakes at Halloween, Thanksgiving, Christmas, Valentine's Day, and Fourth of July. Part of the celebration is donning the aprons, which is always requested by the kids. First, the two oldest grandsons put on white aprons, followed by the triplet grandchildren, two girls and a boy, who ceremoniously put on their red aprons, and then PaPa and JuJu. What fun.

After a trip down memory lane, one can truly see that throughout the generations, aprons have been a tie that binds families together in many ways.

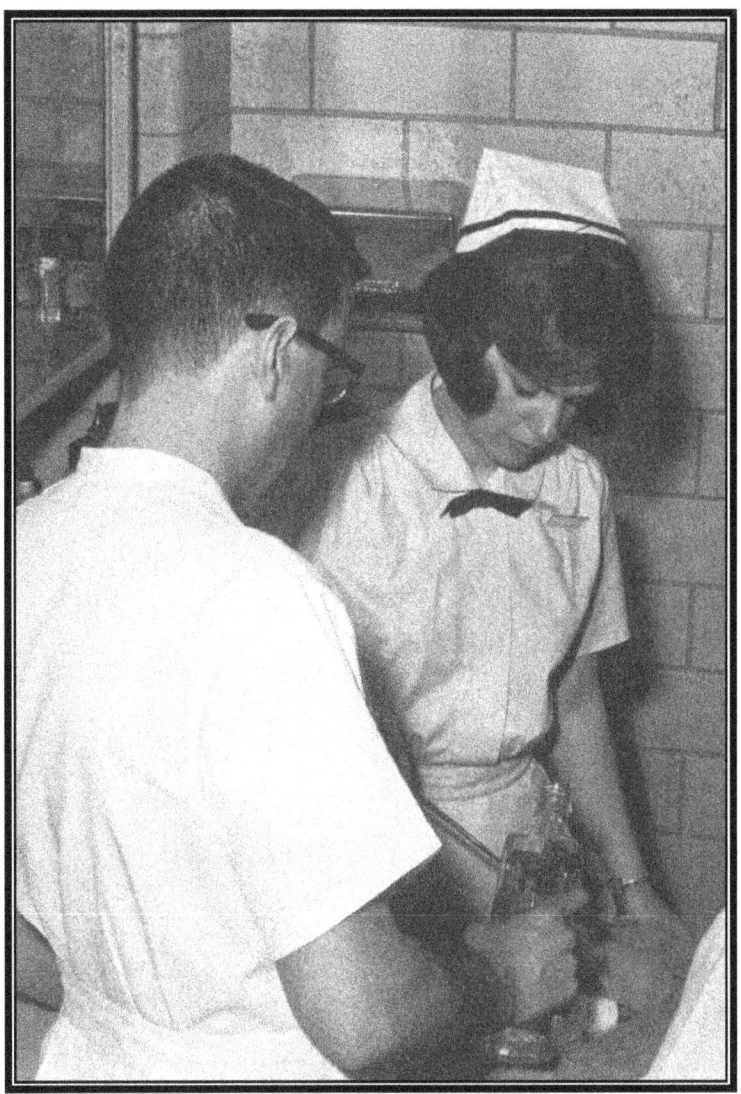

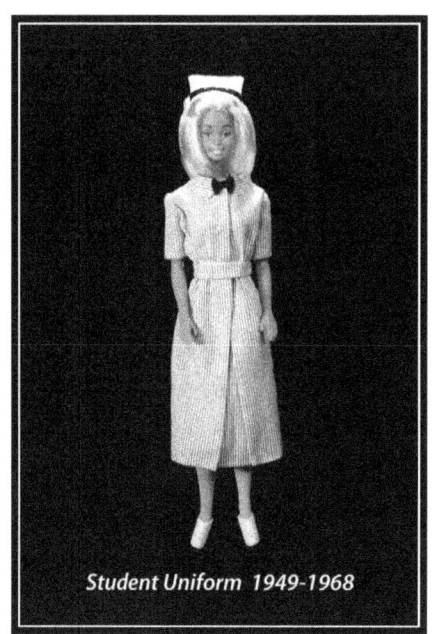

Roy Moncrief was the first male graduate of Vanderbilt University School of Nursing. He and Anne Teutenberg Richardson, both of the class of '66, are shown in the clinical area as students. (photo previously published in the Vanderbilt Commodore, 1966)

Doll dressed in replica of student uniform, similar to that worn by the class of 1966. Image © 2008 Vanderbilt University School of Nursing, used with permission.

Student Uniform 1949-1968

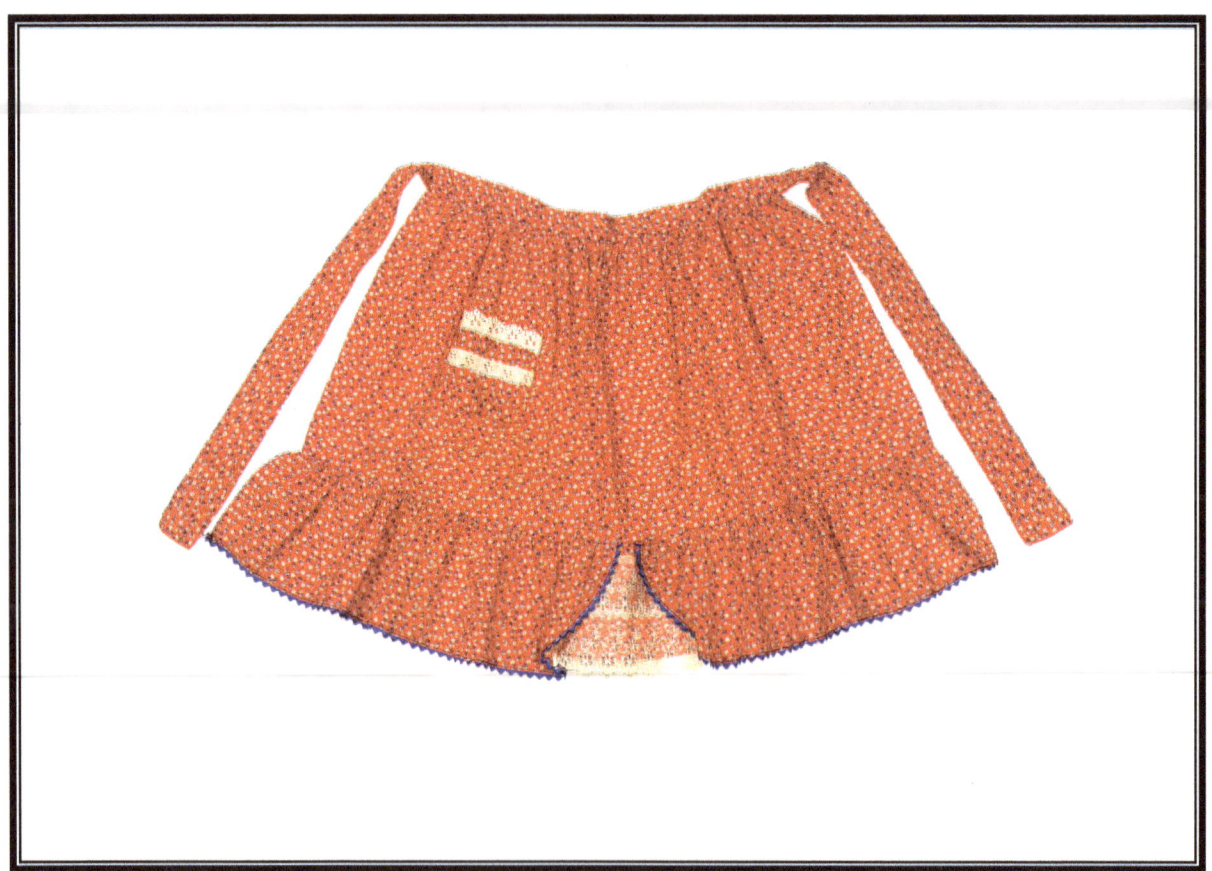

Adopted October 21, 2006 by Sara Jeanne Wells

Sara Jeanne Wells

I am a nurse, as was my mom. She wore an apron over her uniform, but as a student we didn't wear aprons. I personally never, at any time, wore an apron with pockets full of useful things—and the pocket of my adopted apron is too small to hold much of anything—more decorative than functional.

Aprons do conjure up some warm memories and fantasies of domestic bliss. My few memories of wearing an apron may sound sad, but they are really not. Time passes, and how blessed we are to have good thoughts. I remember wearing an apron when my waist was slim, and once upon a time I did have a family to cook and clean for—neither skill my forte, I might add. I was a professional woman. However, having a career first—in time, not priority—and a family second made me appreciate the latter more and an apron somehow symbolized that. Now I am widowed, my children grown with lives of their own. Aprons are reserved for holidays, and today the only aprons I have are holiday aprons, which I pull out for special dinners.

An apron is intended to serve a purpose, to be useful and perhaps to look pretty. They were used for cooking, wiping up messes—people and things—and perhaps to symbolize motherhood and family. But I also wonder—does it symbolize an age gone by? Are we better off now?

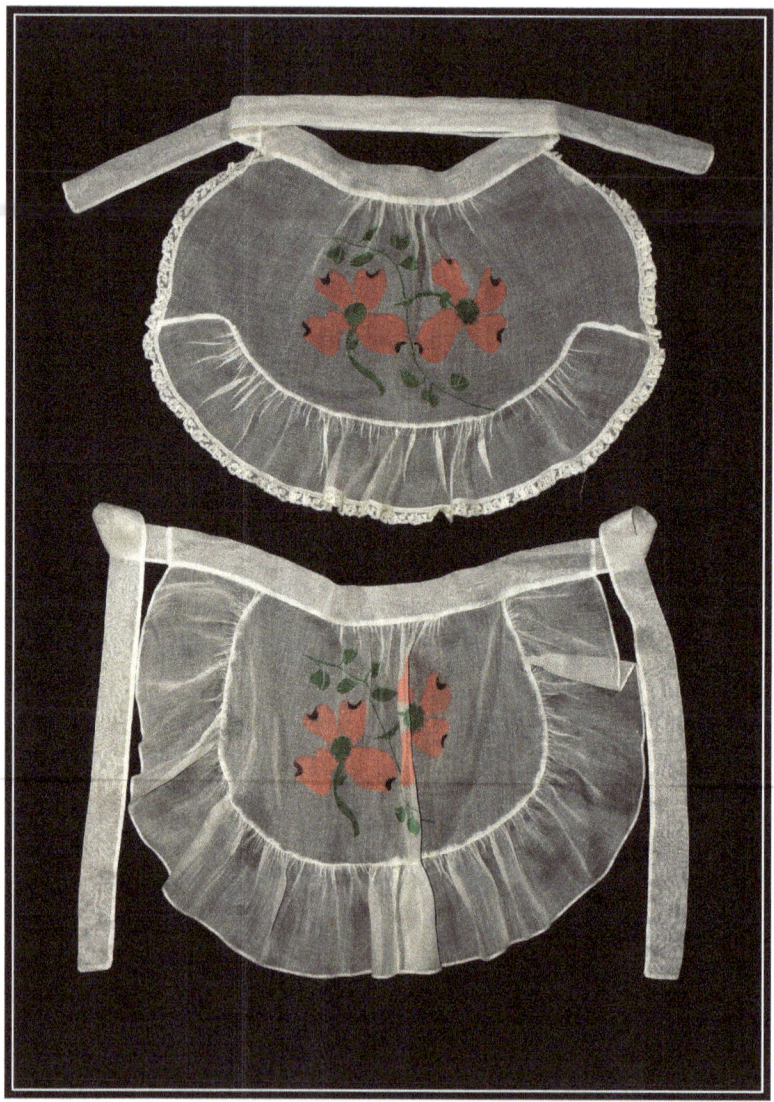

Adopted March 14, 2007 by Amanda Taylor Pendley

A Season

Amanda Taylor Pendley

As we began our busy day
   The sun rushed in to meet us.
      Brought hopes the winter air would fade
         Bring blossoms and new season.

The student asked, "What do you say?"
   With questions from our talk.
      We'd spoke of stages within grief
         The five that come with loss.

She said "I couldn't help but see
   That book upon your desk.
      Forgive my curiosity.
         It's not a nursing text?"

"You mean the one that's leather-bound?
   Oh, no, dear. Tis much more.
      So many answers there I've found,
         Like what you asked before.

When therapy and medicine
   Have done all they can do
      The greatest gift a nurse can give
         Is found only in this book."

We checked our list, prepared to meet.
   The names all looked familiar
      Except for one whose son I've seen.
         Today he wasn't with her.

A Christian widow, always starched
   And bold when she was with him
      Today her eyes had lost their gleam
         Indeed she seemed quite different.

I asked, "My dear, where is your Ray?"
   I dreaded now the answer.
      "Soon God will take my son away.
         He's diagnosed with cancer."

Her salty broken words now pierced
   Our hearts as they were spoken.
      She said, "I don't know what I'll do.
         I've lost my faith. I'm broken.

It's not supposed to be this way.
   I prayed not him, take me."
      The answer given causes blame.
         It leaves me very angry.

She questioned "why" and then she asked,
   "Is God now punishing me?"
      She spoke of things her son had done,
         And those he won't complete.

She spoke of her abandonment
   By father at her birth.
      He left her orphaned soul with fear
         And questions of her worth.

I held her hand and wiped her tears,
   And listened oh so closely.
      The list would have to wait today.
         Her words were too important.

She'd birthed her son into this world
   And held him at her breast.
      She'd nursed him through the worst of times
         Rejoiced when times were best.

No therapeutic plan would come
   To mind so I just listened.
      The sprit took control. "Let's pray."
         Relief came with His mention.

The words spoke of Creator God,
   Who granted each new life.
      Who took lost lambs adopt'd
         For His Son they'd crucified.

I said, "His story now is told
   Like yours in early spring
      But from the loss of earthly life
         Eternal life does spring."

With tears of sorrow mixed with hope
   She left with humble heart.
      She said "I'll do what He commands.
         There's something yet to start."

At end of day, the nurse and I
   Looked back on what we'd learned.
      Reviewed the wisdom and the love
         Our college books had spurned.

She said, "Oh, please excuse my tears."
   I said, "Pray never lose it.
      It's sympathy without the 's'
         It's called the nursing spirit."

On paper now the story sings
   Of mother's love and grief.
      For it was in the early spring
         The apron strings released.

The One who never left her
   Turns blues to pink in masses.
      Sends promise in a sun ray
         And words from Ecclesiastes.

Now each year as dogwoods bloom
   Her tears are mixed with laughter
      As she steps proudly in new shoes
         And speaks of ever after.

To others who have lost their babes
   With tears that can't sustain
      She speaks of One who did the same
         So all could live again.

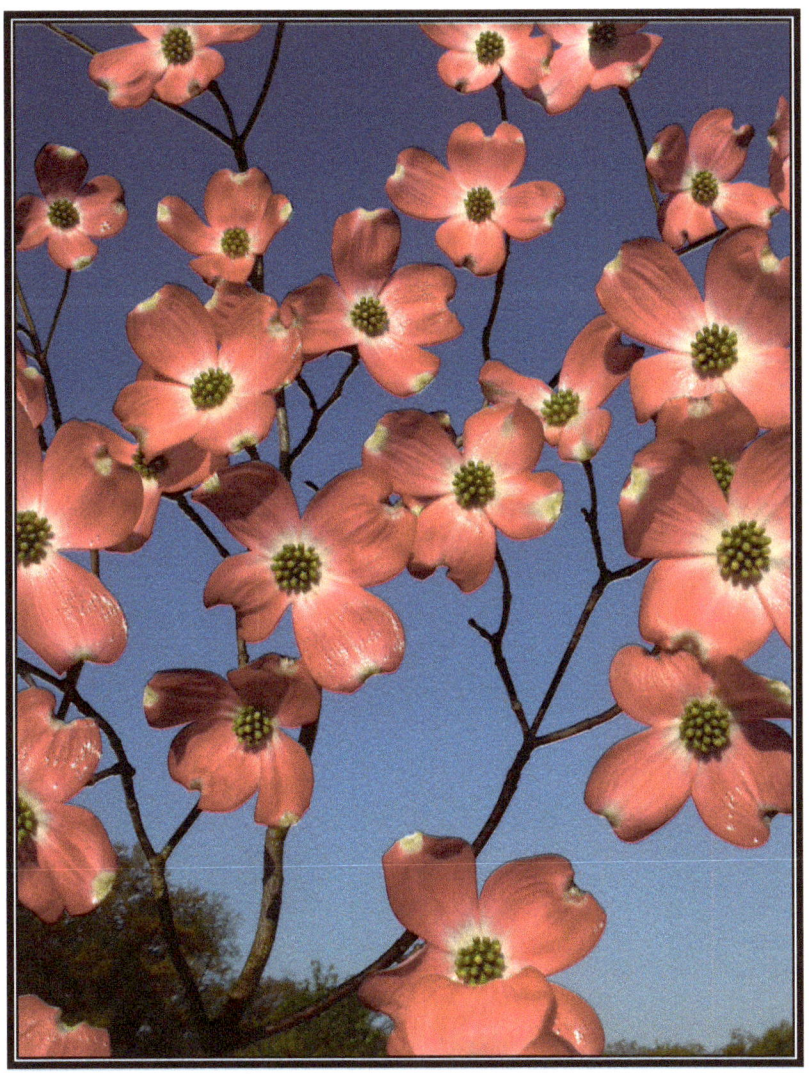

This epic poem recounts a day in Amanda's life as a nurse. Amanda says, "I chose to adopt the two 'mother and child' aprons with the dogwood blossoms on the front, because it reminded me of this true story about a former patient, Ray, who was diagnosed with cancer and was alive when I wrote it, but has just very recently died. It was written in memory of him and dedicated to his mother. Wilma (the bold, starched woman referred to in the poem) asked me to read it at his funeral as part of his eulogy. A copy of the original work, on the dogwood background, has been framed and is now hanging in her home."

Photo by Tom Wortham

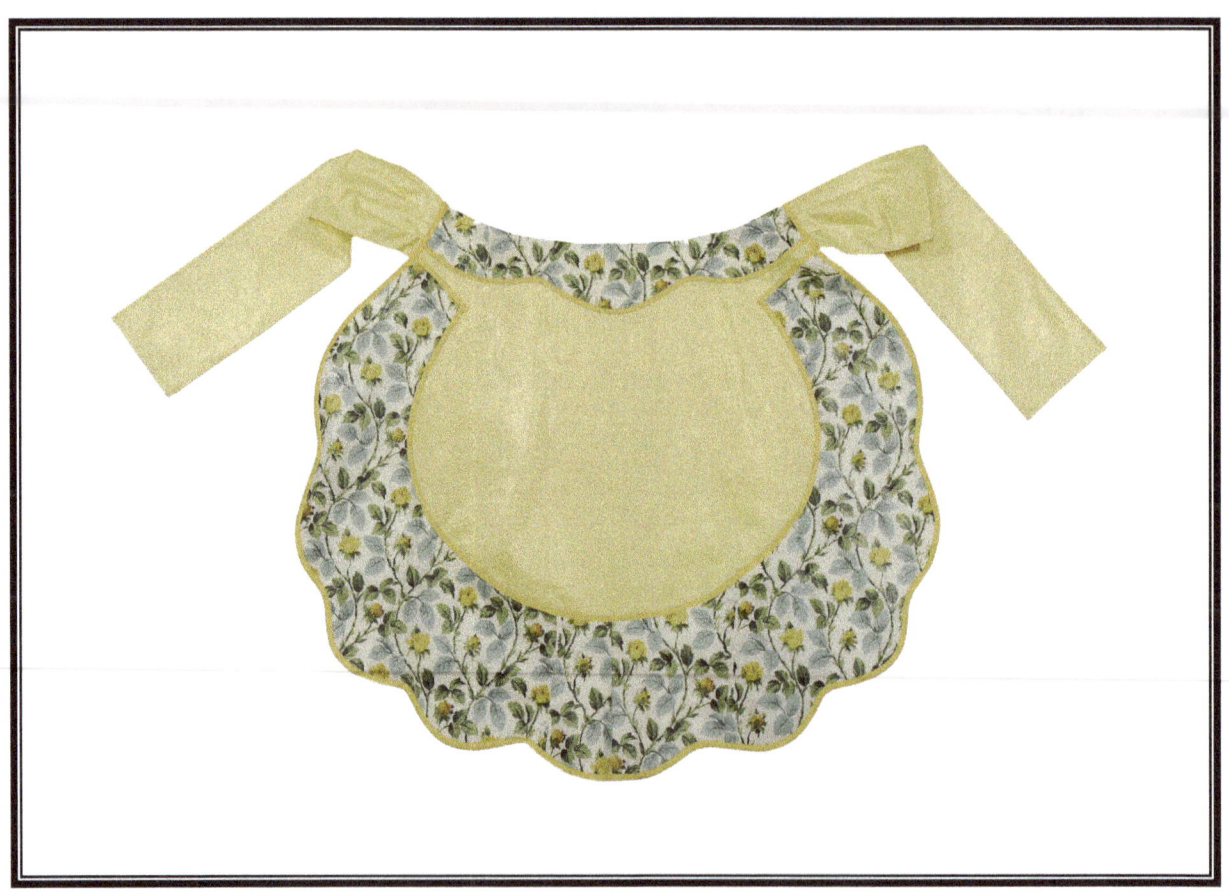

Adopted May 11, 2007 by Rebekah Nesbitt

Rebekah Nesbitt

A four-year-old girl lies in the hospital bed, pigtails in place, still asleep from the anesthesia for her heart surgery. Her small-framed body lies there peacefully, breathing tube in place, with a fresh scar across her chest. Monitors beep, and three nurses are at work settling her in after surgery. The doctors have come by, done their assessments, and left, and the work is now left to the nurses. Each works on a separate task, knowing what needs to be accomplished, and all are aware, subconsciously, of the monitors as they work.

We monitor her vitals closely and get her into a clean bed, then straighten her pigtails and let her parents come in to see her. They enter the room frightened, but relieved expressions soon emerge in their tired eyes. They go to separate sides of the bed, each holding a hand and speaking sweet words to their little girl. They look gratefully at the nurses who have been working—their thanks an unspoken expression on their faces. As the afternoon passes and the parents become more certain that "yes, surgery has gone well" and their daughter is doing fine, more family come in bringing balloons and stuffed animals and a pink princess blanket to fill her bed. The room livens up, and the parents begin telling stories of what their little girl is like; she loves to play with her baby sister, she enjoys being read to, she has learned how to "cook", as she says, and had proudly served her mom Special K and orange juice for Mother's Day recently, wearing a flowered apron. She likes to wear red cowboy boots everywhere. The stories continue to flow. The nurse smiles as she continues taking care of the patient, monitoring everything closely, post-operatively.

As the days pass and the little girl recovers more, the breathing tube and other lines and tubes are removed. For the first time, the nursing staff begins to see the girl, about whom we have been hearing, emerge. They are there—the red cowboy boots, the flowered apron, and all.

For all of the ups and downs that nurses endure as we work in so many different capacities, this is why we do it—to be a part of the miracle of giving children a second chance, or helping a mother make it to her son's thirty-fifth birthday, or helping a baby born too early learn how to feed and thrive. Though it can be sad and stressful at times, we are privileged to enter into so many lives and to share compassion and love, as we work to help patients and their families heal and cope. It is a call to service, but one that comes with many rewards and joys, and one that can be filled with stories of little girls with aprons who will be able to continue living their four-year-old dreams.

GOTCHA COVERED: A LEGACY OF SERVICE AND PROTECTION

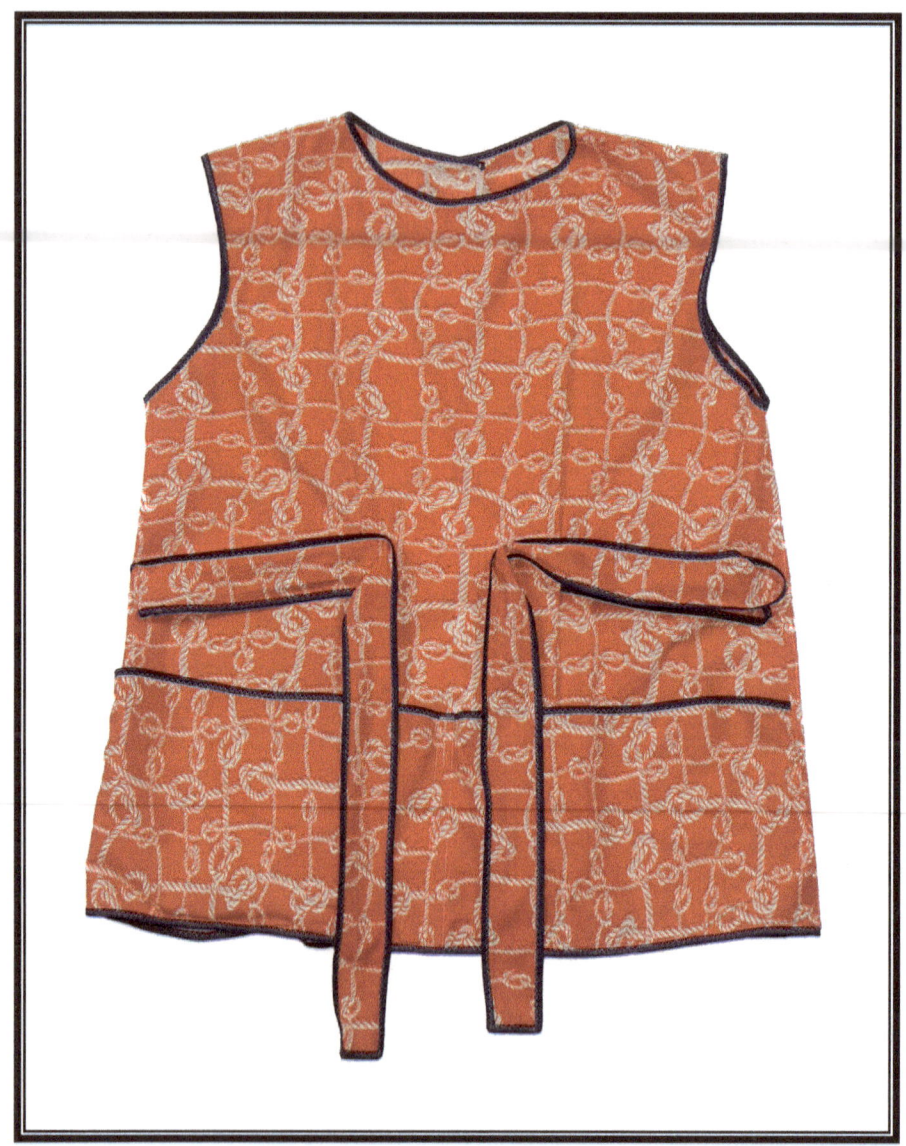

Adopted April 4, 2009 by Susan Kaburu

Susan Kaburu

The first apron I wore was in 1973, when I was a student nurse. The aprons were fastened by a safety pin, which was on our nameplates. The apron was for protection from spills and direct contact with dirt and splashes when performing nursing duties, such as sluicing, turning patients, and bed-making. After qualifying, no more aprons were needed, as we were assigned to administrative duties. These days, aprons have been replaced by gowns. To me, aprons indicate noble service, as they are worn by those in various service professions. It represents a calling, in that you are doing willingly for others something that is messy and can cause anything to happen to your clothes, but all the same, you respond. It also reminds me of the towel Jesus used to clean the feet of His disciples.

GOTCHA COVERED: A LEGACY OF SERVICE AND PROTECTION

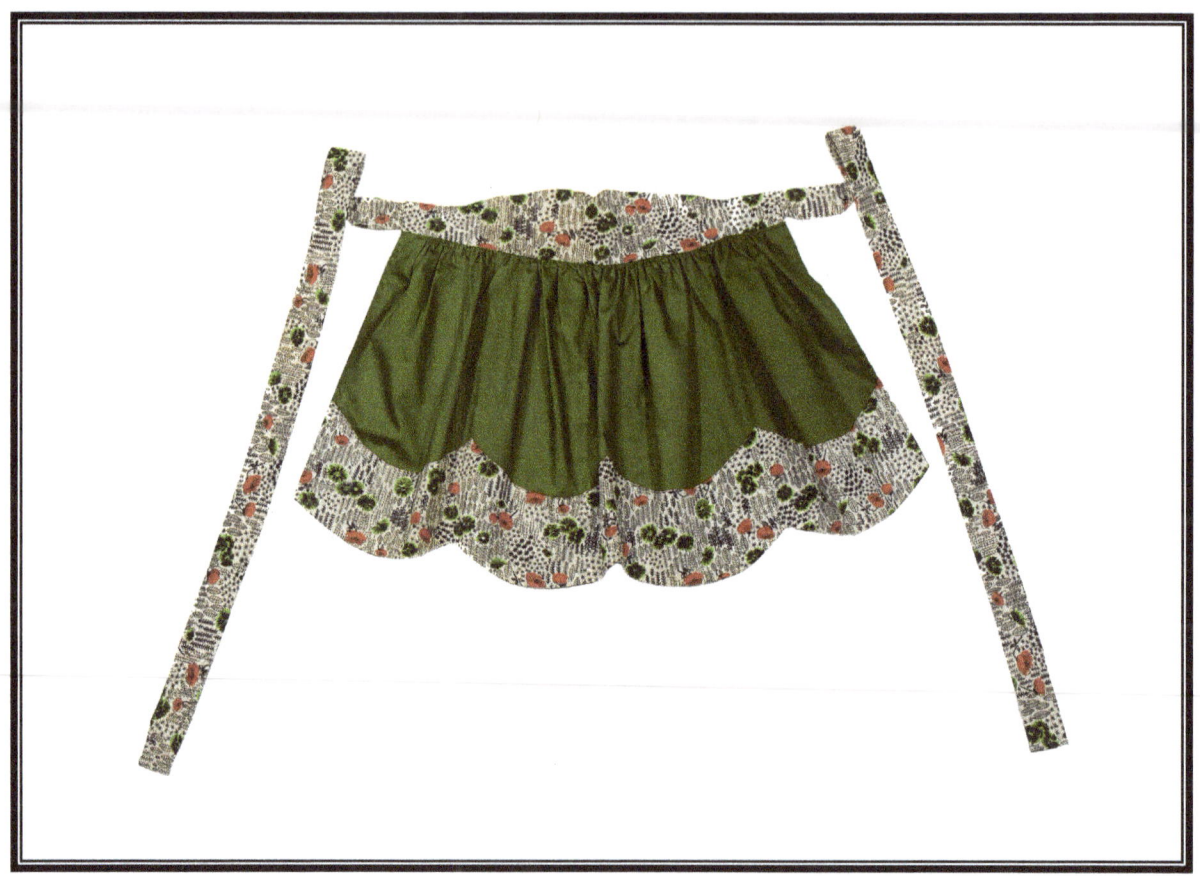

Adopted January 31, 2007 by Virginia M. George

Virginia M. George

I have only worn one apron in my life. I wore it only because it was required for me to reach an important goal in my life. That apron was the white, unattractive, long apron that covered the equally unattractive, green nursing uniform at Vanderbilt University School of Nursing. My goal was to earn the BSN degree in nursing, which was accomplished in December 1947. Wearing that apron was worth what it helped me achieve.

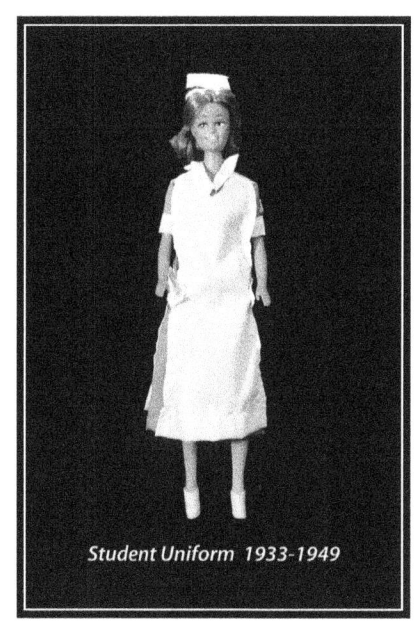

The student uniform worn by Virginia George
was similar to the replica on this doll.
Image © 2008
Vanderbilt University School of Nursing.

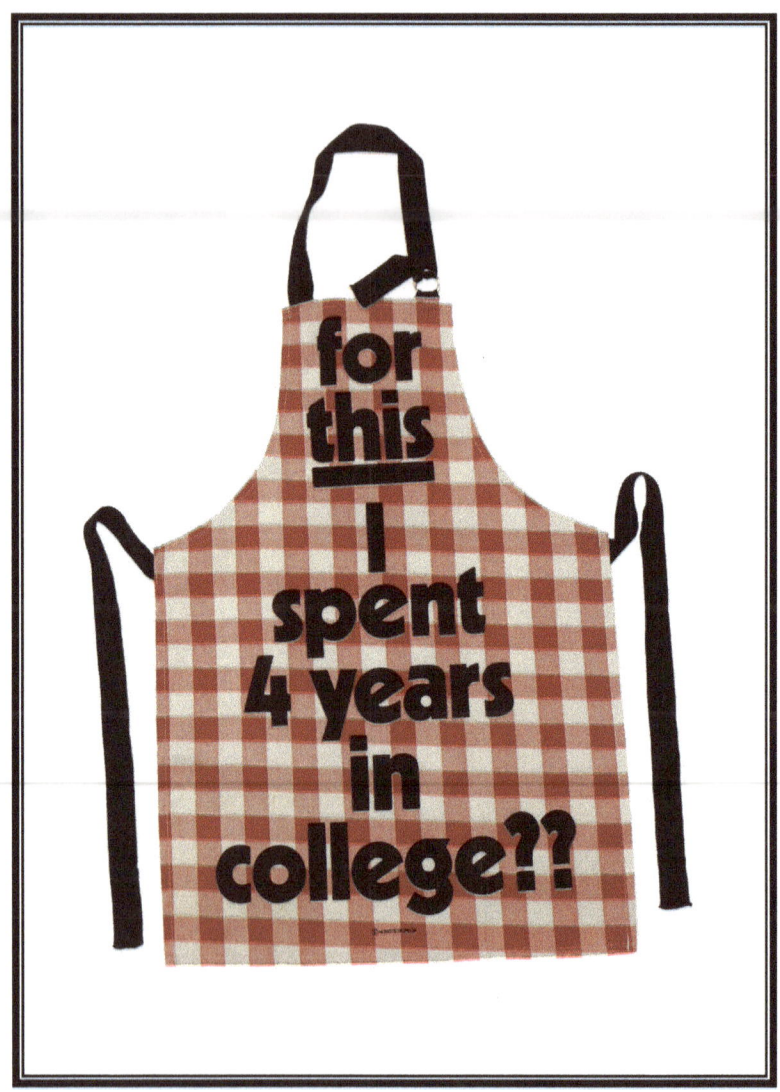

Adopted March 14, 2007 by Brooke Faught

Brooke Faught

Nursing is rarely the sterile, excessively gratifying, and heroic profession that is represented in the media. In reality, nursing often involves many of the competencies of medicine, without the same respect or recognition that physicians receive. Many nurses, including myself, made their nursing debut as a nurse's aide. Others stumbled into their first clinical experience wearing starched uniforms or scrubs, shiny clean shoes, and immaculately groomed hair. By their second day, their uniforms or scrubs and their shoes probably had stains, and their hair was simply fastened out of the way without concern for style.

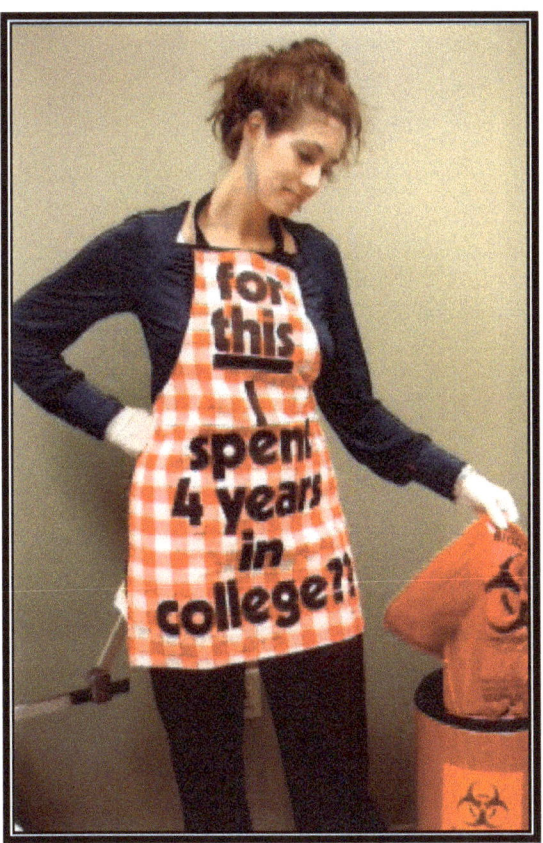

This is where the true nursing experience began. This is where the nurse learned that it's not about the recognition. It's much simpler. As simple as the whispered "thank you" from a patient for providing a bedpan, for giving a sip of water, or for offering a reassuring word.

No, nursing is not a glamorous profession, but it is a magnificent one.

Brooke humorously illustrates her essay with this image of herself wearing her adopted apron.
Photo courtesy Brooke Faught

GOTCHA COVERED: A LEGACY OF SERVICE AND PROTECTION

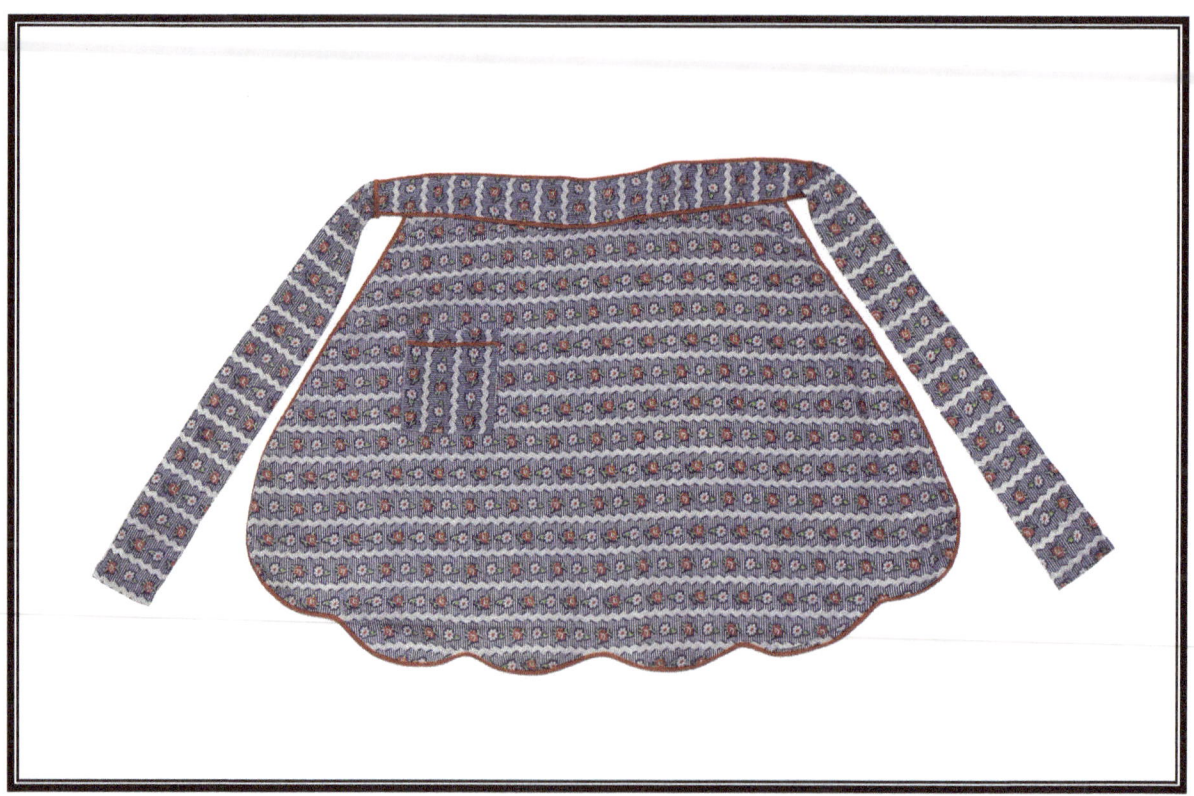

Adopted November 18, 2006 by Cynthia Fielder Diamond

Cynthia Fielder Diamond

I was attracted to my apron because the colorful, flowered print reminded me of the everyday dresses my grandmother sewed for me when I was a little girl. Those dresses, meant for play, were made from fabric reclaimed from cloth sacks that held huge amounts of white flour. My grandmother used the flour to bake delicious biscuits, cakes, and piecrusts. After the bag was empty—and the cheerful cotton sacking washed and pressed—there was just enough material to sew a child's dress. Each time a new bag of flour was delivered to my grandmother's home, I knew that I would soon be given a new outfit.

In the fall of 1950, I began first grade—at that time there was no kindergarten or preschool in rural Tennessee. My flour-sack play dresses were put aside in favor of school dresses. School clothes were sewn from plaids and ginghams purchased at the local dry goods store on the town square or, most prized by me, ordered from the Sears and Roebuck catalog. I already knew my teacher and many of the children in my first grade class, so I was most fascinated by that group of students who came to school by bus. These new friends lived on outlying farms, had squeaky new shoes, and the girls wore dresses made from flour sacks. I could not fathom why they wore play clothes rather than school clothes, but thankfully I asked no questions. However, in my snobby, town-child way, I felt knowingly superior.

In the fall of 1962, I came to Vanderbilt University. Vanderbilt is physically located only one hundred miles from my home, but at that time, it was culturally much more distant. During my freshman orientation, I became aware that my entire college wardrobe was not in fashion. The stylish coeds wore madras wraparound skirts, oxford cloth blouses, and Villager sweaters. I wore print dresses made by a local seamstress and skirts and sweaters purchased at Sears and Roebuck. I thought of the flour-sack dresses lovingly stitched by my grandmother and I wished for one to wear—at least I would have been thought of as unique rather than frumpy. My classmates in the school of nursing never commented on my wardrobe, but remembering my feelings of superiority toward those first-grade farm girls, I wondered what they really thought. A few new friends helped me shop. My parents sent extra money. By spring semester, I also wore madras and oxford cloth.

The next year, as sophomore student nurses, we were fitted for our school of nursing uniforms, and we were allowed to care for hospitalized patients. This uniform was both unstylish and unflattering, but I loved it as much and wore it with as much pride as I wore those flour-sack dresses sewn by my grandmother.

PART TWO: *Aprons as Symbols of Identity and Service*

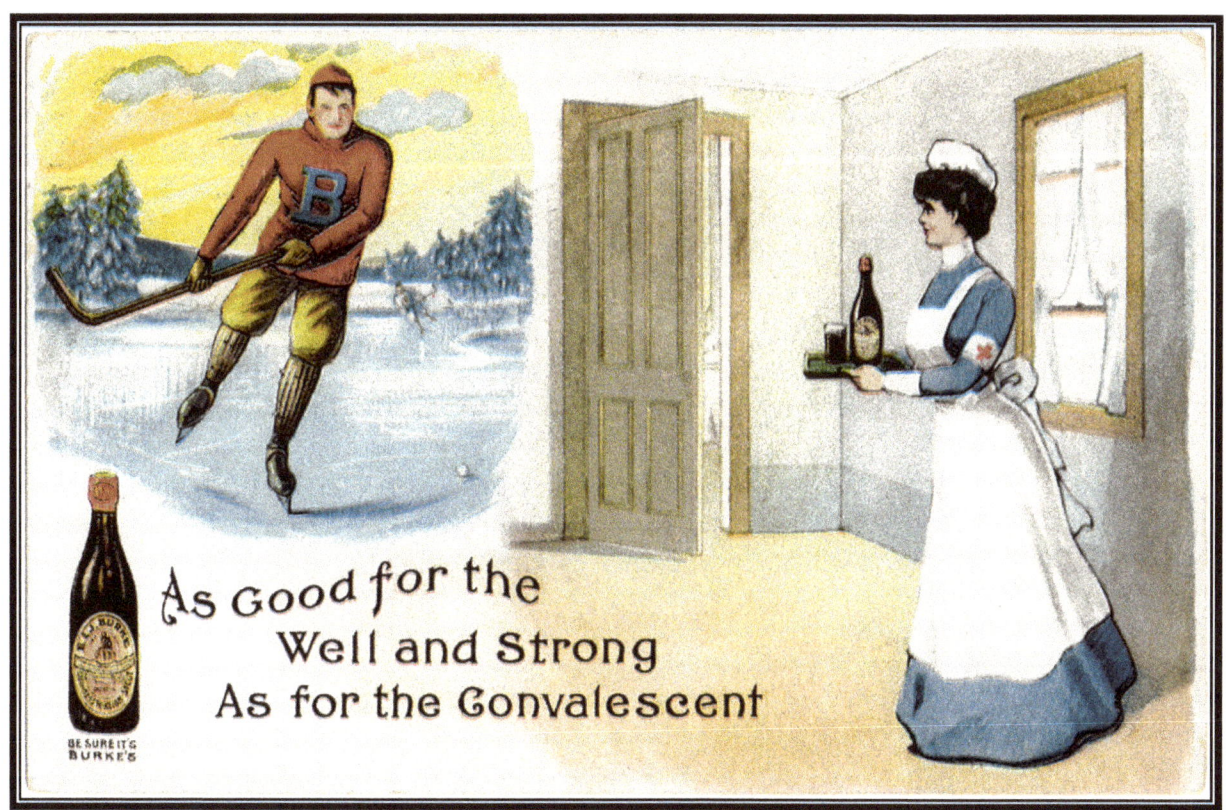

© Zwerdling Nursing Archives, used with permission.

Aprons as Symbols of Identity and Service

Ginger T. Manley

When I put on my aprons the children mind me better, wandering visitors immediately know my role as a stay at home mom. Door to door religious missionaries assume I am a virtuous woman and cheerfully move on to the next house. Fred thinks I look cute as a button, and neighbor children hug me more often.

Hillbilly Housewife, posted at www.hillbillyhousewife.com

Humans have probably used some form of the apron since the time we began to wear clothing. "Throughout history, sexuality, politics, social behavior, religion, gender, and love have been conceived, controlled, and corrupted by a small piece of cloth, sometimes plain, sometimes embellished, always significant," comments Maine author Cynthia Thayer. (Cynthia Thayer, e-mail message to Ginger Manley, May 23, 2009)

Aprons have historically been used to cover and protect, to convey membership and identity, to symbolize service, and to carry items. Indigenous people covered their genitals with apron-like cloths to protect themselves from injury or exposure. In Genesis, God tells Adam and Eve to cover themselves with an apron, or in some translations a fig leaf or loincloth. Another Biblical passage describes the symbolic power of aprons in the service of healing. "And God did extraordinary miracles by the hands of Paul, so that handkerchiefs or aprons were carried away from his body to the sick and diseases left them and the evil spirits came out of them." (The Holy Bible, Acts 19:12)

By the Middle Ages, certain groups of male tradespeople had become identified by the aprons which they wore as part of their work. Freemasons wore leather aprons which provided pockets for stowing tools and which protected their midsections as they handled heavy stones. Other tradesmen like shoemakers, blacksmiths, butchers, carpenters, gardeners, tailors, clock makers, painters, furniture makers, and bakers wore aprons for the same reasons. When an apprentice was promoted to full status, he received an apron to signify his position. Shopkeepers donned aprons as symbols of their roles, as well as to protect their clothing from the often dirty work of hauling and stocking their wares.

Medieval housewives had few dresses, and they protected what clothing they had by wearing aprons, which covered their clothes almost completely. Different classes of women wore aprons of different materials and color. Poor women wore aprons of rough, hard-wearing fabric in a natural brown color. Middle-class women wore linen aprons dyed blue, which was a favorite color for wearing to church. Wealthy women, who had the luxury of time, often embroidered their aprons, but even these were never that elaborate. Since aprons were a badge of respectability for proper women, it was a rule of society that London's prostitutes were forbidden to wear them.

In eighteenth-century England, a woman could not transfer ownership of property to a spouse, but such was the powerful symbolism of aprons that the term *apron-string tenure* came into existence. Such tenure allowed a man who married a woman who had property to use it while his wife was alive even though he did not get title to it. Since such a man was in no position to protest his place, the phrase *tied to her apron strings* came to stand for any event in which a man had to submit to his wife or mother.

Over time, ceremonial aprons became a part of our culture. By the eighteenth century, aprons had become symbolic of fraternal membership for Scottish Rite Masons, whose history links to the medieval Freemasons. George Washington's Masonic apron illustrates the level of intricacy in the design of such symbolic aprons. Mormons have traditionally employed a fig-leaf-adorned apron for all temple-worthy members. These ceremonial aprons are worn as part of their temple endowment ceremony. Most faithful Mormons and Masons are also buried in their symbolic aprons.

After Queen Victoria ascended the throne and had her official portrait made wearing an embroidered apron, such aprons became the rage in England and elsewhere. By the mid-1880s, black afternoon-tea aprons were *de rigueur*. Following the death of her husband, Prince Albert, the queen always wore black, and late-nineteenth-century women wore black mourning aprons along with other black dress in solidarity with her, to signify their bereavement.

While almost all women of this era wore aprons as part of their dress, "(t)he various aprons worn by working-class women were usually functional items made of serviceable fabrics. There was a marked visual contrast between the parlour-aprons worn by the ladies of the house and the aprons worn by the parlour maids who waited on them." (Smith, 2003, p.13) Highly collectible, vintage aprons from this period show intricate, hand-sewn embroidery done by women as a statement of their upper-class social standing, indicating they had time available for doing such art.

The mid-eighteenth-century styles of nurses' aprons not only provided coverage where spills might occur but served as literal vehicles for transporting all manner of necessities. Georgy Woolsey, one of two sisters who became nurses during the U.S. Civil War, has been described as, "(e)ver alert for ways to make patients more comfortable and their care more efficient, she kept her apron pockets filled with forks, spoons, corkscrews, and other useful items." (Stein, 1999)

Over time, wedding aprons have been worn by brides as either cultural or religious symbols. Modern brides sometimes wear functional wedding aprons to prevent getting their wedding dress soiled during the reception. One contributor to this anthology remembers a pre-wedding ritual in 1966:

> *On the night before I was married, after the rehearsal dinner and while I was getting ready to spend my last night in their home as a single woman, my parents gifted me with a beautiful white organdy and lace apron, which was ceremoniously tied on me by both parents. My parents then simultaneously pulled out a pair of hidden scissors and cut the apron strings, hugged me, then handed me the apron and the ties.* (Suzanne Blievernicht, e-mail message to Ginger Manley, December 2, 2006)

By the mid-1800s, middle- and upper-class girls wore decorative aprons, called pinafores, as part of their clothing for both casual and more formal occasions.

By the end of the nineteenth century, women's aprons not only protected their clothing, but also identified their employment roles. Nurses, nannies, and housemaids were easily recognizable in their similarly designed, full-wrap aprons, usually accompanied with a frilly hat. Early twentieth-century schoolteachers, waitresses, shopkeepers, and others wore aprons both as objects of identity and for protection over their clothes. In rural areas, aprons were made from whatever was on hand, in many cases feed and flour sacks. For many people who wore aprons as part of their employment, the apron often had multiple functions in addition to covering clean clothes and identifying the trade. They were frequently used to gather and carry items like wood from the shed, or eggs from the coops, or vegetables from the garden.

People owned relatively few items of clothing until recently and what clothes they had needed to last a long time. Washing was a tedious process, and it was easier to keep clothes clean by covering them with an apron than to change their clothing frequently. Our ancestors often owned more work aprons than clothing, and they wore full-bib aprons of differing fabrics and styles for many tasks. A handbook for salespeople in the 1920s has detailed information on sales techniques to induce women customers

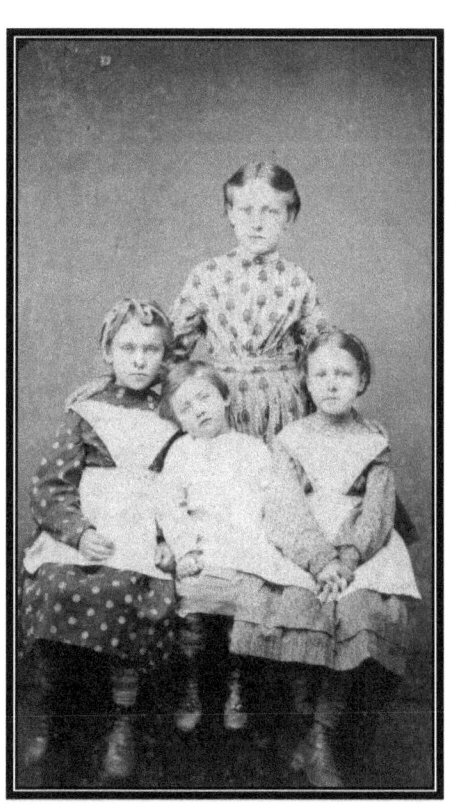

Smith children in pinafores, c. 1856.
Photo courtesy
Manley family archives.

to buy a variety of aprons along with their new dresses. (Kneeland, 1925) By the 1950s, with the advent of electric washing machines and synthetic fabrics, it became easier to keep clothes clean. When women began to own a wider variety of clothing, there was less need to cover them, so the half-apron became the apron of choice. The fabrics and designs of that time indicated that women wanted their aprons to be fashion accessories more than utilitarian items.

For the postwar woman, aprons were symbols of both territory and ownership, and of her domestic role in service to her family. Almost every person born before 1970 sees June Cleaver, in her apron and pearls, as the quintessential housewife of the era. Images of apron-wearing mothers were prominent in children's literature from the late 1950s until the 1970s, and little girls were often gifted with apron costumes, which they could wear to become imaginary apprentice housewives.

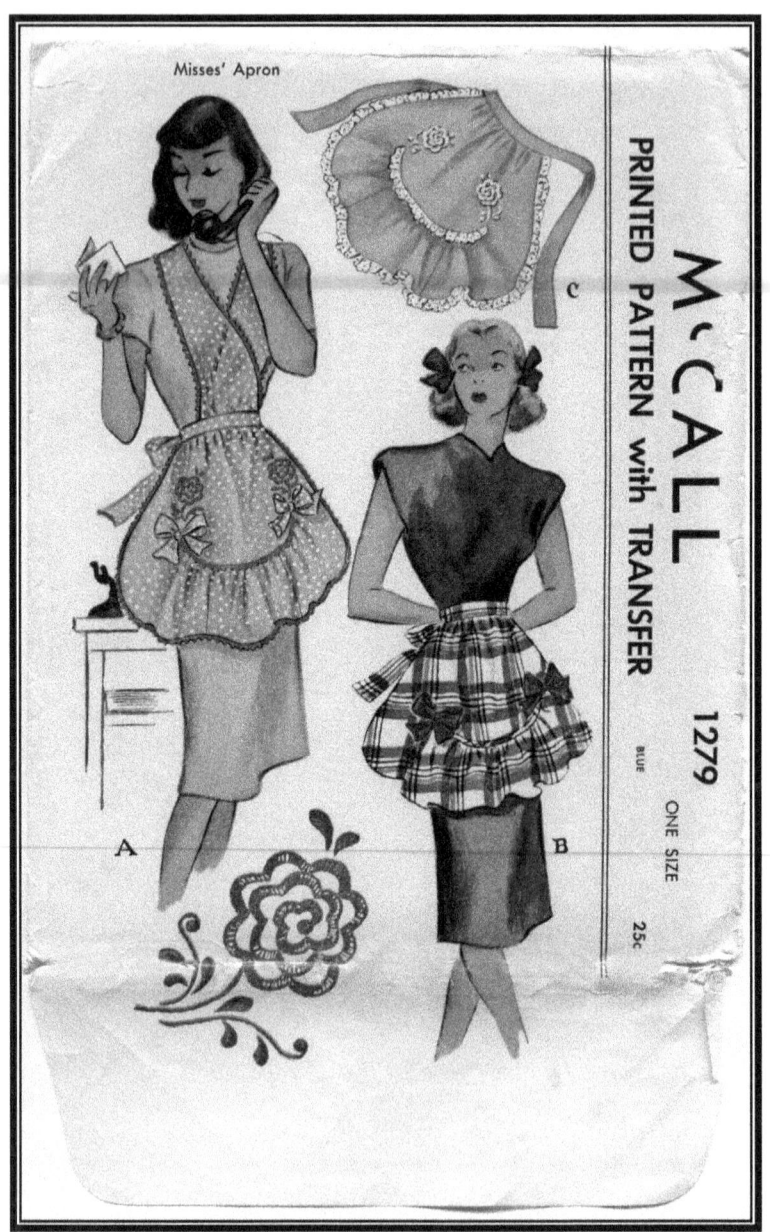

McCall pattern #1279 © 1946 McCall Patterns. McCall/ Butterick Vogue Pattern Company, used with permission.

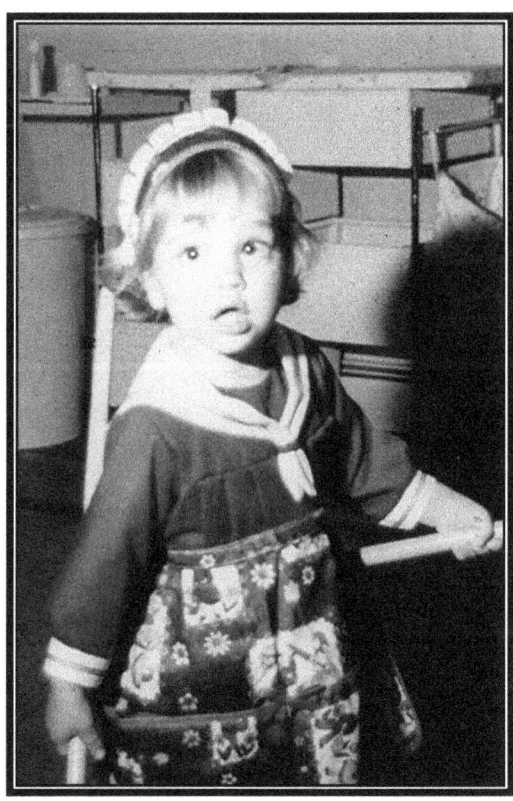

Elizabeth Manley, c. 1969, costumed as an apprentice housekeeper.

Elizabeth Manley (now DeWerth) grew up to major in math in college and now works from home, raising three young children and writing interactive college math textbooks. She rarely wears an apron in either of these occupations, but she voices fond memories of wearing this apron in her childhood. Photo courtesy Manley family archives.

In the children's book, *Apron On/Apron Off* (Scholastic Book Services, 1968), Joan, a kindergarten-age child, learns from her parents about the roles aprons play in society for both men and women. However, after trying on various apron-clad roles as baker, newsboy, shoemaker, and printer—all characterized as males in the story—Joan ultimately ties on her child-size half-apron and joins her mother in cleaning the house.

Several scholarly papers examined the role of aprons in portraying stereotypical mothers in children's literature. Linda Oliver (1974) presents a list of desirable female images for elementary school readers, including "all mothers do not wear aprons." (p. 255) Lois Rauch Gibson (1988) compares the negative, stereotypical, and caricatured apron-clad mother-depictions to those positive ones of archetypal mothers in children's literature, concluding that some authors "may go beyond the apron in a variety of ways." (p. 177) According to Gibson, the Mary Poppins character illustrates both a stereotypical and an archetypical woman. Mary "is versatile and surprising, like her own carpet bag, out of which come her apron, a large cake of soap, a toothbrush, a folding chair, a cot, all of Mary's nightclothes, and various and sundry other things." (p. 179)

In late-night reruns of *The Andy Griffith Show*, filmed in the 1960s, Aunt Bee is the apron-wearing mistress of her kitchen. She even gives up the lead in the town play to return to the kitchen and tie her apron back on when her rival, Clara Anderson, moves in to tend to Andy and Opie in her absence. In another segment, Aunt Bee has just left the house in a twitter, wondering whether her boys will survive her three-day absence. Andy closes the door and gently nudges Opie toward the kitchen to face a sink-full of dirty dishes. Both head straight to the aprons draped across the counter. Opie puts his apron around his waist, crisscrossing the ties around to his front to tie them. Andy puts his on, tying it (badly) in back. Then he lovingly stoops to reposition Opie's apron, which is now grazing the floor. Andy unties it, raises it up under Opie's armpits, allowing the apron to cover all the territory between Opie's chest and knees. Both boys turn to the dishes—Andy washing and Opie shaking the still-wet saucers in the air to remove the water, before stacking them in Aunt Bee's corner cupboard. The message is clearly that they are awkward visitors in Aunt Bee's territory, even if they are wearing aprons.

The apron's place in culture changed in the 1970s, when it became symbolic of servitude rather than service, and powerlessness rather than empowerment. When liberated women discarded their aprons, they believed they were flinging off domestic enslavement. If these liberated women owned aprons at this time, the apron usually served as a vehicle for conveying a protest message.

By the 1990s, aprons started to reappear, first in the form of barbecue aprons or as gourmet culinary fashion for both genders. Women who grew up in the '50s and '60s were drawn to aprons because of a nostalgia fueled by mellowing. Younger women, who had no prior identity with aprons, were coming of age and trying to reconcile their harried status with what they perceived to have been the less-busy experience of their mothers and grandmothers. Many of these women began handcrafting and scrapbooking in groups with other women as ways to invest in themselves and each other, and they started wearing aprons, something that they had probably never seen their mothers wear.

By the beginning of the twenty-first century, a full-fledged apron revival was occurring in the United States and abroad. Web sites and blogs devoted to apron trivia and crafting sprang up. Apron exhibits, sometimes with extensive curating, began to occur in this country and elsewhere. In South Australia in the late 1990s, Avis Smith studied the apron as a vehicle of "cultural technology in which and by which women were trained into certain roles of femininity, domesticity, sociality, and passivity." (Craik, 2006) Joyce Cheney published *Aprons: Icons of the American Home* (Running Press Book Publishers) in 2000, after extensively exhibiting her apron collection in museums across America. Her carefully documented, historical accounts and photographs of aprons offer a fascinating view into both vintage and modern aprons. EllynAnne Geisel toured the United States for seven years with her Apron Chronicles, an exhibit of aprons, apron-inspired stories, and photographs. She published *The Apron Book: Making, Wearing, and Sharing a Bit of Cloth and Comfort* (Kansas City: Andrews McMeel) in 2006, and established a national "Tie One On Day," occurring the Wednesday before Thanksgiving. The first "National Wear Your Apron Day" occurred in 2008, planned to occur annually on the Monday after Mother's Day.

In early 2009, *AARP The Magazine* ran an article about surviving the current financial recession. The magazine used two artist renderings of modern-day women in their homes wearing 1950s-era, frilly half-aprons to illustrate the concept of frugality. (Kirchheimer, 2009) During the same month, the e-zine, *Smart People*, posted a summary of a major research study done at Cornell University and published in the March 2009 *Psychological Bulletin* (Ceci et al., 2009). The research analyzed thirty-five years of evidence on why "math-proficient women are underrepresented in math intensive fields." (SPmag admin, 2009, p. 1) In the online article, titled "Apron Strings Keep Women Out of Math Fields," the phrase *apron strings* is used as a metaphor for childrearing and other domestic responsibilities of women. The reported research concluded that women who enter math-intensive fields often drop out before they advance, by necessity choosing domestic and nurturing roles over an advanced math-related role, a choice that almost no men are forced to make.

For some of the contributors to this anthology, the apron symbolizes service in the best meaning of that word. For others, the apron evokes memories of servitude and restriction of autonomy. These are powerful symbols to be represented by such a humble garment.

IDENTITY LEGACIES

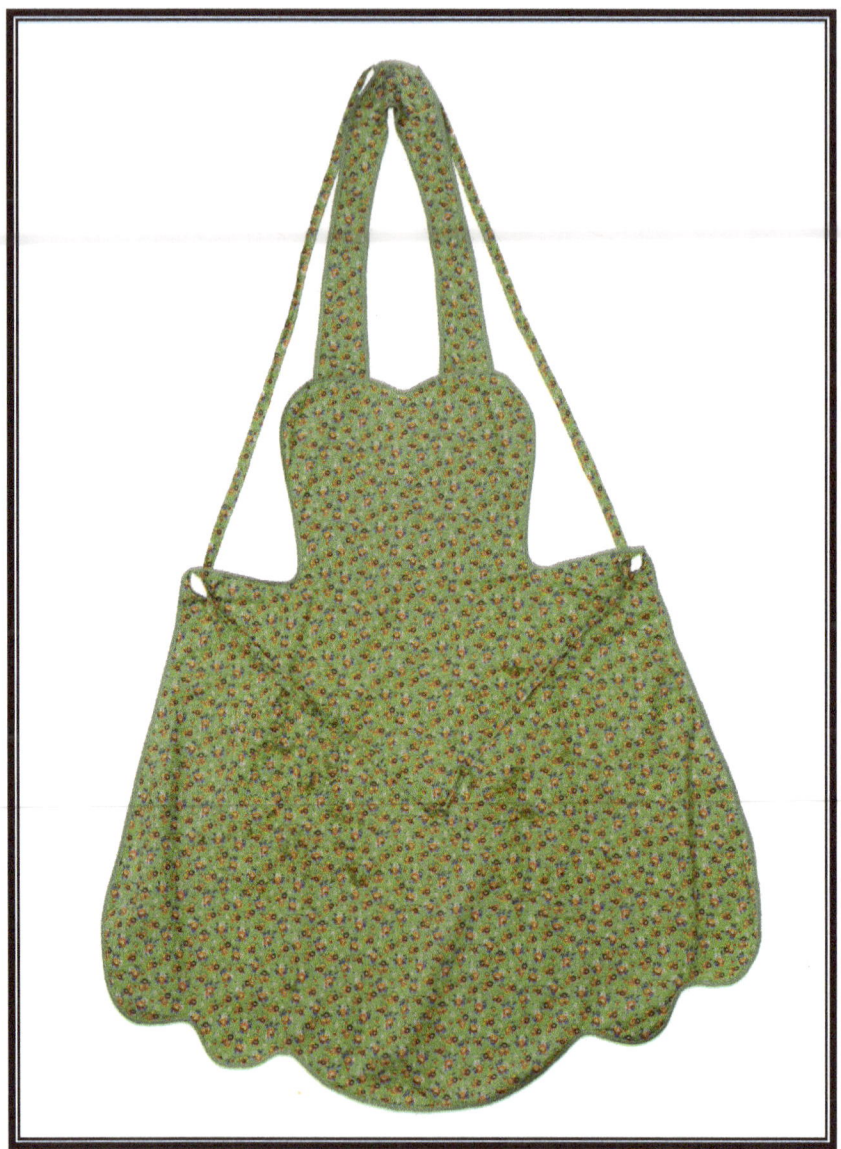

Adopted December 20, 2006 by Carol Etherington

Apron Remembrances

Carol Etherington

Aprons are for remembering
        Busy hands and smiling faces now at rest
        After lives lived long and well.
Aprons are for remembering
        Places filled with messy, flour-covered children and
        An abundance of mirth.
Aprons are for remembering
        Times gone by that will never come again.
        But oh, how lovely the memories.

Gotcha Covered: A Legacy of Service and Protection

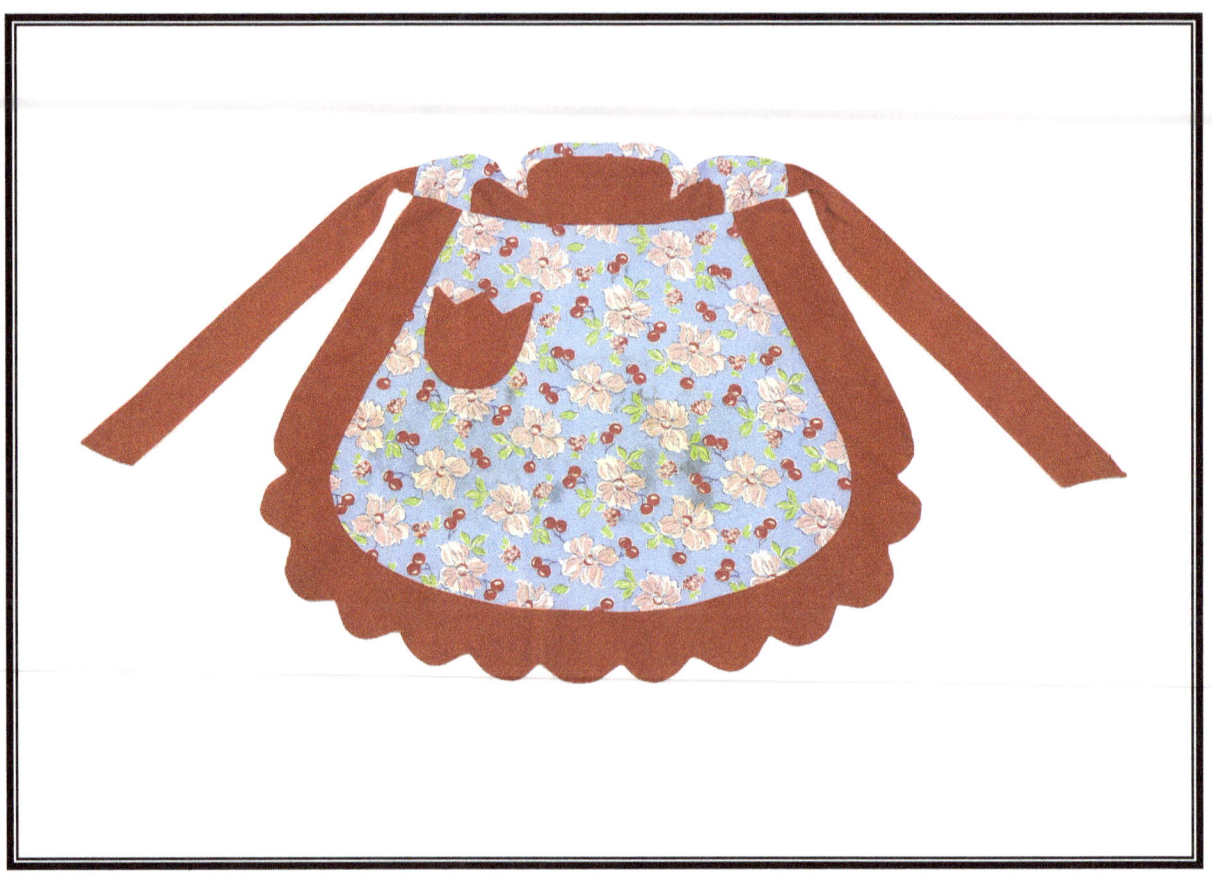

Adopted October 28, 2006 by Marti Mueller Daniel

Pressing Matters

Marti Mueller Daniel

When I was young, I used to read my mother's hands as a sailor reads semaphore flag signals. Her hands were not just body parts attached to her limbs, but two separate spinning aggregates, independently gesticulating, directing, claiming, discharging, and fluttering. They appeared to act and react before cognition, before linear thought. With an anticipatory flair of "something's coming," her hands gathered up her apron, snapped the fabric decisively, and then sliding down the ties, took them with calm certitude around her waist to her back. She quickly tied a bow and gave a sharp yank on the loops to indicate that she was on the edge of diving in.

We lived in a small, two-family, brick duplex. Everything had a place and a way of being. In the ship-shape nature of our first-floor flat, whatever could not be physically labeled became verbally designated, and being so named, never changed. Monikers like The Towel Drawer, The Apron Drawer, and The Coat Closet were called out like longitudes and latitudes during our daily activities. These labeled-and-named keeping places became part of our family lexicon. Hands-on and tangible, they felt safe and secure.

A much different world existed down in the belly of our basement, a stone-gray grotto, dark and mysterious and scary, where two large furnaces inhaled black coal with a fire-red mouth. Going down there took nerve. The concrete floor and steel support posts, eerily lit by a series of tiny street-level windows, made the day seem like night. The edges of *self* dissolved with each step on the creaky, open, wood stairs, requiring a rapid metamorphosis of internal systems, from nerves to blood, from the conceptual to the purely instinctual.

I loved it.

At the foot of the stairs was a loosely described area that we called The Laundry Room. I often followed my mother up and down the stairs, perching myself on a low step to watch her work. We were Demeter and Persephone, playing out our own mythology as we traveled back and forth between the upstairs kitchen and the subterranean underworld. Every week my mother gathered the laundry and descended to the basement, where cotton piles flowered up, encircling the round electric washtub with its hand-cranked roller wringer. This work was not for the weak or the careless. It involved chemicals and heavy equipment, and a faith that things once blemished or broken could again be restored. As the seriously stained clothing soaked in a bleach solution in the sink, she swirled starch into a small bucket of water.

Out in the yard, she spun a white clothesline between the house and the garage, creating a veritable web just waiting to catch an unsuspecting prey, wet and fresh. Using hands, arms, feet, legs, and even her mouth, into which she would place two or three clothespins at a time, my mother scuttled down the rows like a spider, weaving back and forth, all limbs in action, one eye on the sky, one eye on the task. When it rained, the clothesline crossed the landscape of the basement, and the air was moist and heavy from the dripping wash. On these days, her sunny side-step movements were replaced with a soulful dance of slower rhythms, her body shifting intuitively into sidereal time, silent and distant. The day was internalized, and the whole basement was transformed into a white labyrinth of excellent hiding places.

Washday was pedestrian, however, compared to the painstaking protocol and ritual of ironing. After the stiff and puckered laundry came off the line, rewetting the material was imperative for a fresh finish. I watched my mother's hand dip lightly into a small bowl of water, her fingers flinging droplets sharply down over each piece of laundry as it was anointed, gathered into a ball, and gently congregated in the basket. The radio was turned on, the ironing board unfolded, and the electric iron set on *High*. At that point, as if to claim advantage and dominion, my mother raised the heated iron with her right hand. Swiftly, she touched the bare flesh of her left middle finger to her tongue and aimed her moistened finger fearlessly toward the iron's silver base. The hissing ping of this volley and her skilled rapid rebound was nothing less than high art.

I wanted in.

In the heat of this desire, my mother and I forged a female bond. She taught me how to hold and pass the iron over flat cloth with my right hand, and how to use my left hand to pull and tug the material taut. In no time, I was accepted as an apprentice to iron my father's large, plainly hemmed white handkerchiefs and her more delicate hankies embellished with crochet and embroidery. I loved the smell of the wet cotton as the water molecules gave way beneath the pressure and heat of my iron. The steam that rose up from the fibers was infused with a sharp tang of detergent and bleach; delicate hints, redolent of the atmosphere, drifted up from an earthy and deep base, the origins of which were rooted at one time in a field, someplace warm. I breathed the steam and felt satisfied, at peace with the geometry of it all.

I passed the iron along invisible vector lines stretching from corner to corner, I arced the iron in a semicircle back and forth, and I enjoyed making crisp creases. I loved to see the handkerchiefs stack up on top of each other, little folded pancakes just waiting for syrup. I learned the differences between fathers and mothers as I put the handkerchiefs away in their respective dresser drawers: scattered loose coins versus jewelry boxes, horse-racing forms versus perfumed sachets, abandoned leather wallets versus silk scarves.

When I graduated to ironing the aprons, however, the tidy squares and rectangles gave way to ruffles, puckers, pockets, pleats, long ties, and various grades of fabric weight and sheen. My straightforward formulas no longer applied. I faced multiplicity. I debated with myself. Was it better to iron the waistband and ties before the skirt? Would the crinkled tie open to the approach of the iron without my other hand getting in the way? Should I iron over the top of the gathers or nestle into each one? Every damp apron was an uncharted map, all directions fluid and free. With my undomesticated tenacity, I navigated their borders. Resounding from them was the language of kitchen, of garden, of dinner party, of holiday, of art project mess and protection, hers and mine.

Over time, I learned how to stay in the moment without rushing the finish. Between the apron and me were spaces and folds, fabric and flesh. I made friends with transformations, and sudden and inexplicable mishaps; I straightened things out; I soothed wrinkles and crumpled edges. I began to learn how to maintain fullness.

Pressing forward toward a future of challenge and difference, feeling my way around the double seam of burden and *jouissance*, these early aprons lay down as colorful bridges upon which I could move from inside to outside myself, and beyond.

Meditatively, unconsciously, I began to grasp with two hands not only the apron as object, but also myself, a conversing female subject, joining the visual, tactile, and olfactory sensations with which I was engaged to the very fiber of my being.

Gathering up my basket of finished work, I would climb the basement steps, returning to my mother who was setting the table.

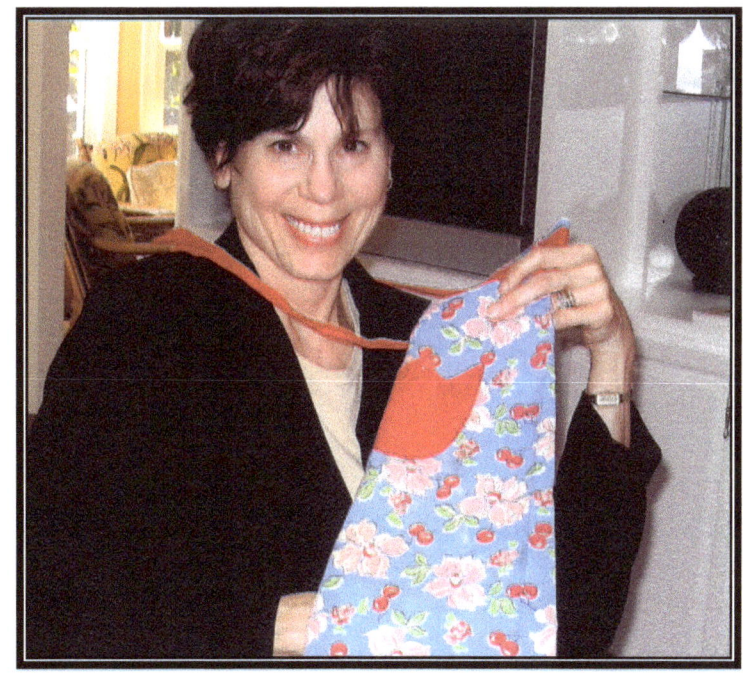

By the time Marti returned her adopted apron to the collection, she had formed a strong bond with it. Photo courtesy Manley family archives.

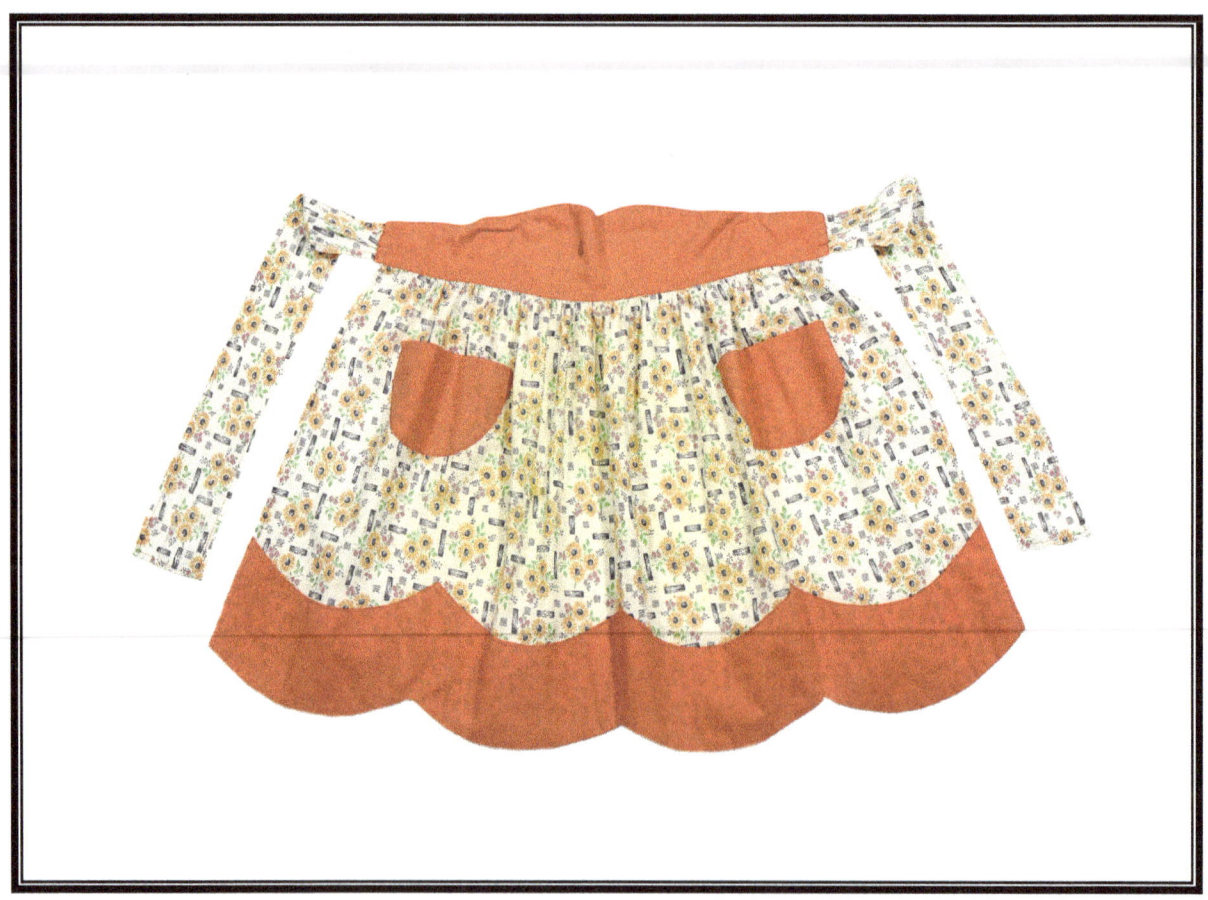

Adopted April 6, 2007 by Mary Gresham Buchanan Barr

Apron Tribute

Mary Gresham Buchanan Barr

home·ly - /hom li/ Pronunciation Key - (**hohm**-lee)
Adjective -li·er, -li·est. 1) Lacking in physical attractiveness; not beautiful; unattractive: *a homely child.* 2) Not having elegance, refinement, or cultivation. 3) Proper or suited to the home or to ordinary domestic life; plain; unpretentious: *homely food.* (*American Heritage Dictionary*, Third Edition)

Through a series of events, including a tenant who skipped out on several months of rent, I once found myself with a cat and a green restaurant apron. The cat was black and white. The apron was the type with a bib that can be worn around the neck or folded over. The straps were long enough to cross in the back and then tie in front. The pockets were deep and the tie in the front could hold a hand towel. I found myself starting to wear it if I was baking and didn't want to get flour on myself. Meanwhile, I got married, moved across the country, and started having babies, moved back and finished having babies. The green apron lived through it all. The cat went to heaven.

Recently another apron made its way into my life. The orange color is jarring in its repeat at the waistband, the pockets, and the large scallop. The tan flowers fade against so much orange. From the picture I have, the material is spotted and thin, shiny from repeated use. If I were to see it up close, I might wonder if the seams are wearing. It is, in fact, a homely apron.

I wonder about the way we use the word *homely*. Why does a word with the lovely root, *home*, have such a different use as an adjective? The most common usage, *unattractive*, gives as its example "a way to describe a child." As if any child could be ugly. The second most common usage continues the lack of respect; "not having elegance, refinement, or cultivation." It is not until the third usage that the glimmer of hope begins for the word and for the apron.

As a teenager in the 1980s, I shunned the apron and all I thought it represented. June Cleaver, with her pearls, heels, and apron, vacuumed constantly and waited for everyone to come home. No thank you. As a new nurse working nights, I ordered a pepperoni and jalapeno pizza every third day or mooched at my parents' home, coincidentally coming to visit at mealtime. When I met my husband, I laughed when I learned that he had eaten a meat and two vegetables every night throughout his time in medical school. As we started dating, I found myself cooking more and more. He was literally so exhausted as an intern that one evening he fell asleep in his plate of mashed potatoes, broccoli, and chicken.

I might have been cooking almost every night, but no way was I wearing an apron.

Babies do not grow up on pizzas alone. My now fifteen-year-old son and thirteen- and eleven-year-old daughters would love to return to the pizza days, but I am now quite a cook, with a rotating supply of restaurant aprons in various colors. As I wrap the ties of the apron around me, I find the plain domestic activities of preparing dinner, settling disputes, and listening to the day's details are not sophisticated or glamorous, but "plain" and "unpretentious." It is, however, a very rich and blessed time in my life. My apron is an integral part of service and love for those in my life. My adopted apron was an integral and much loved part of another woman's life and kitchen, enabling her to serve others. No apron can be "lacking in physical attractiveness" if it is being used in the service of love and care for others.

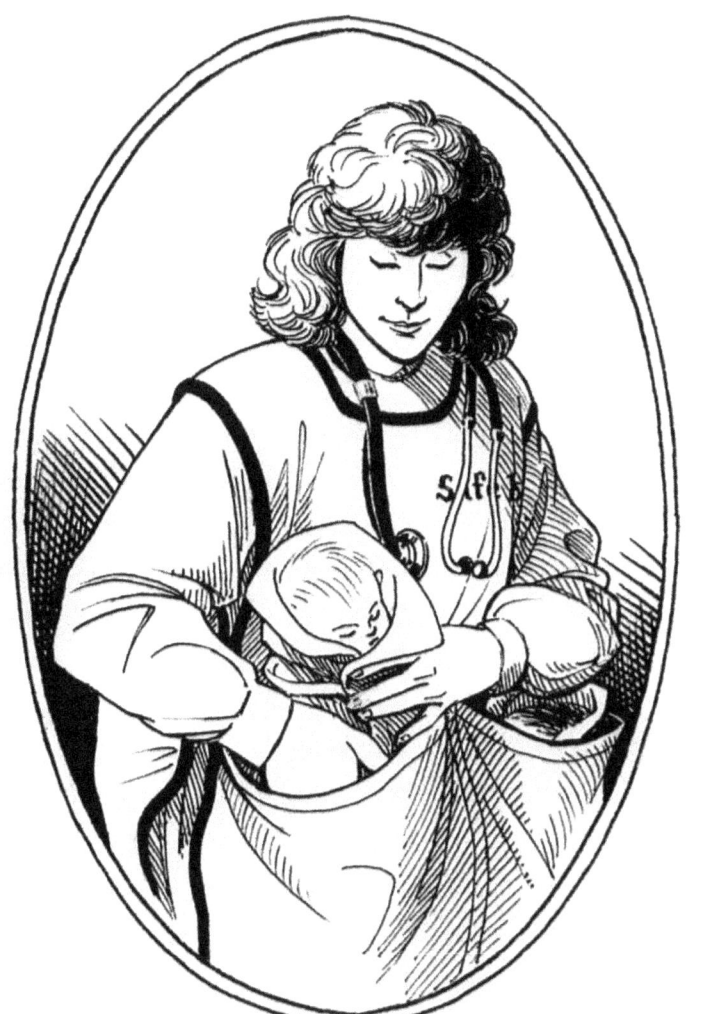 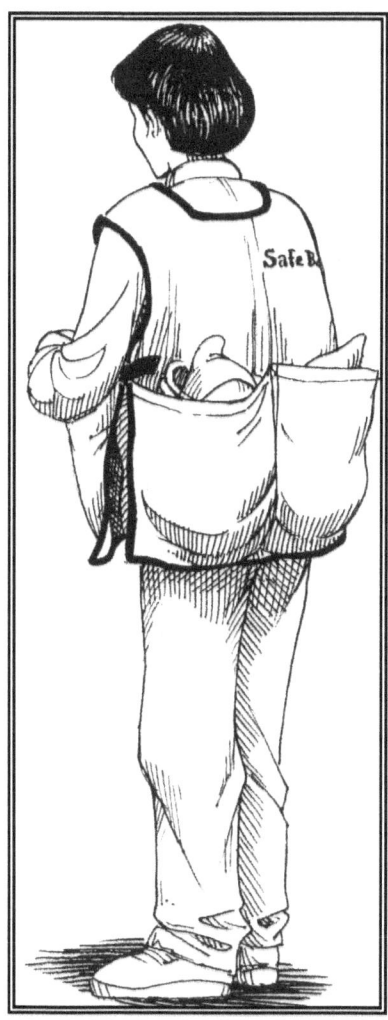

These illustrations show a modern evacuation apron used by neonatal nurseries and other child-care facilities to safely carry four swaddled babies per apron in the case of an emergency. While protecting the infants, the nurse's hands remain free to maneuver as necessary. This is a marvelous example of a twenty-first century nurse's apron which is both for service and protection. Safe Babies infant emergency evacuation aprons illustrations courtesy of International Health Resources (www.SafeBabiesAprons.com).

GOTCHA COVERED: A LEGACY OF SERVICE AND PROTECTION

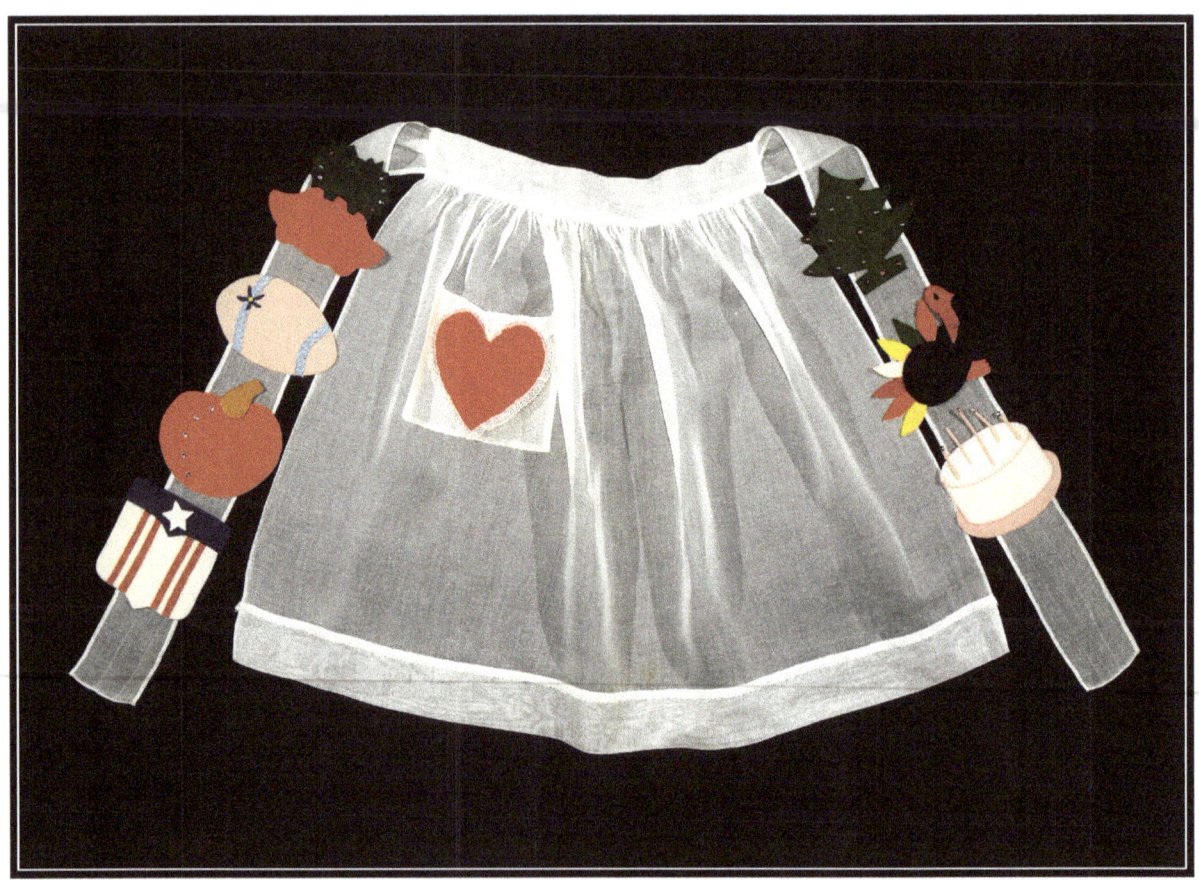

Adopted October 21, 2006 by Ginger T. Manley

My Apron, My Self

Ginger T. Manley

How is it possible for me to have apron nostalgia or, more correctly, *euphoric recall* of apron times when I have spent my adult life, as a woman and as a nurse, being apron-defiant? I did not want my life, domestic or professional, to be defined by an apron tied around my waist, so I own only one apron—well, actually two. One is a sturdy, canvas, bib-type affair bought in a shop in the New Orleans airport about fifteen years ago as a gift for someone, and then kept for myself. It covers my front well when I remember to wear it, which is about half the time that I am cooking, so it has the requisite stains from greasy handprints. Not the Crisco kind of stains of my ancestors, however—not in today's health-conscious world where olive and canola oil are the shortenings of choice.

The other apron is a souvenir from the Viking Culinary School class I attended last year. I had quite ably prepared meals for my family for more than forty years using the most basic of kitchen implements, but to my amazement, some of my friends made a big deal about specialty cheese graters, six-burner gas ranges, and $175 roasting pans. To satisfy my curiosity, I signed up for the *Tuscan Dinner Party* class, where I was given a brand-new, white bib apron to wear as an apprentice chef. Working in a small group of three—in a larger class of twelve led by a young woman chef—we learned to make biscotti, and osso bucco with gremolata and risotto, and broccoli rabe. Then we sat down and ate—no, devoured—our creations, and we were awarded the aprons we had worn during the class as our graduation presents. I have never worn that apron to actually cook in my own kitchen. It is "too good to wear."

Which brings me to the vintage aprons in my inherited collection. Being "too good to wear" has allowed almost fifty aprons from the '40s, '50s, '60s, and '70s to survive into the twenty-first century. My family was practical. They survived five generations of rural, East Tennessee living, including losing the family farm during the Depression. My parents' generation fought in World War II, then coming out of that, they brought solid middle-class values to American society in the 1950s as I was starting to grow up. Meals were prepared from scratch, often from fruits and vegetables grown in our own garden. For a while, eggs and chickens from our own backyard brood kept the table supplied with scrambles and fried chicken. By the late 1950s it was easier to get meat and fowl from a grocery or market, so the coops were dismantled and replaced with a huge outdoor cooking place, fired by hardwood or by charcoal depending on the menu for the night. Backyard cookouts took place here with my dad wearing a chef's apron.

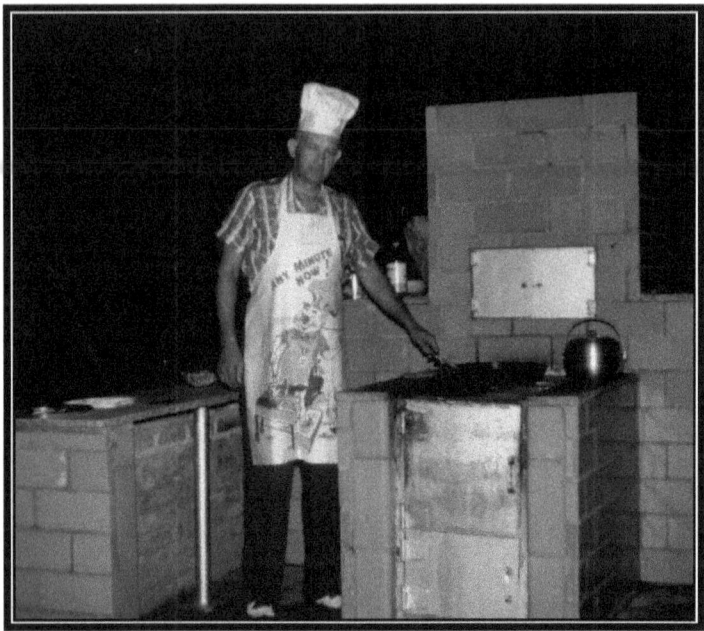

Scott Trundle,
proprietor of the outdoor grill, c. 1960.
Photo courtesy Manley family archives.

My mother, also, always wore an apron. She put on an everyday apron for breakfast and housework, and then in the late afternoon, she changed to a clean-up-in-the-afternoon dress and a better-looking apron. Never a fancy one, just sturdier chintz or calico for getting the supper meal on the table. The apron did not come off until after the supper dishes were put away and the last flour-sack dishtowel was hung up to dry.

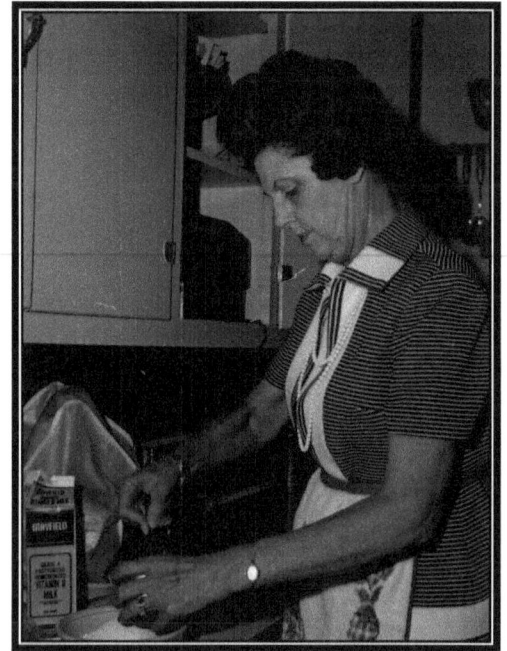

Alice Trundle,
proprietor of the home kitchen, c. 1962.
Photo courtesy Manley family archives.

There were, however, other aprons—ones fashioned especially for parties. For these special gatherings, the apron was as much a part of the festive dress as the faille skirt or the sweetheart neckline of the summer dress. Party aprons were usually organdy or polished cotton—crisp fabric which could be starched to hold its shape. They weren't expected to actually absorb spills from a ten year-old's toppled-over Kool-Aid or to wipe up the smears from a chocolate-frosted cupcake. These were the ones that were "too good to wear" for everyday use.

I have changed my mind about aprons. They no longer represent being chained to domestic slavery. As a friend of mine recently remarked about herself, "I got my feminist, anti-establishment, women's liberation stuff out of my system about the time I hit menopause." Aprons were intensely personal for my ancestors, a symbol of ownership I now understand. My mother owned her kitchen when she was wearing her apron. My father owned the grill when he was wearing his apron. I don't have any memories of such domestic ownership in my own adult life, and I am poorer for the void. I have adopted a vintage apron from the collection of fifty or so that my aunt had carefully folded away in a chest of drawers. And I am richer for the opportunity.

Today my adopted apron is wearing a heart, but it comes with ten other snap-on, themed pocket patches. At Easter, I can change to a pink, decorated, Easter egg snap-on. For any of the Federal holidays, there is a white, breast-pocket-shaped snap-on, sporting vertical red stripes with a blue chevron smartly crossing the top of the pocket, and set off in the middle by a white star. There is a snap-on, white birthday cake decorated with pink frosting, holding five pink candles, their tips glowing with pink sequins. Thanksgiving has a brown turkey with multi-hued tail feathers and a red gobbler head. Halloween has an orange pumpkin. Christmas has two options—a sequined, green, Christmas tree or a doublet of red bells with green holly-leaf handles. Thank goodness this apron was "too good to wear" and survived into my late life. It is a priceless treasure of who I am and from where I have come.

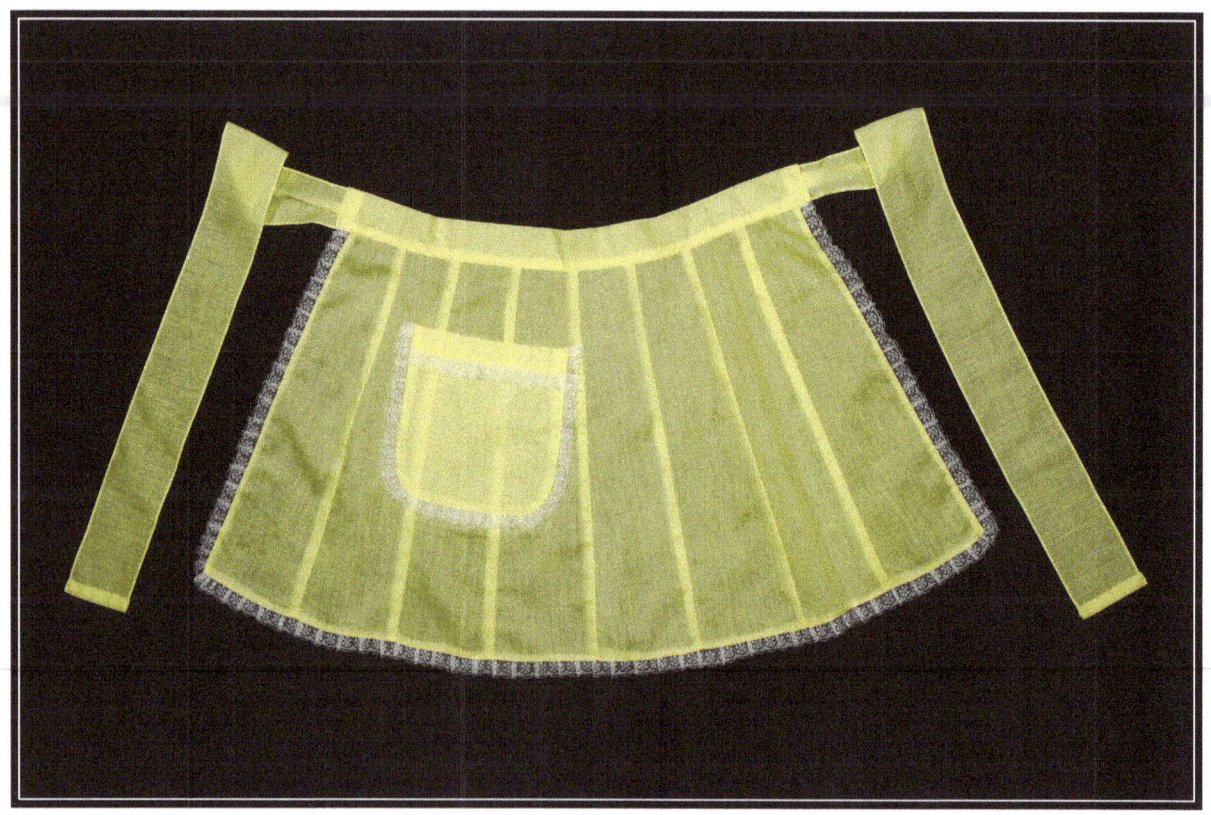

Adopted May 17, 2007 by Diane Carlson Evans

Judge a Woman by Her Apron! Not!

Diane Carlson Evans

Behold the sight of Aprons!
There will soon be cookies out of the oven. Hurrah!
Or is it pies? Even better!
Or, onions out of the garden!
Is that flour or dirt on her apron?
Oh, I do hope it's flour!
My lovely adopted apron isn't anything like the utilitarian aprons used in our home during my childhood. Dainty "Adoptee No. 13," in its elegant, yellow organdy, finely lined with lace and sweetness, would not have suited our domestic duties during those years. However, I did see *her* at wedding receptions, funeral luncheons, and teatime in my auntie's home. But, no. Never at the Carlson homestead on Rural Route 3 in Buffalo, Minnesota. Life there was close to the earth—no time for fuss or frills. I would never have worn an apron "just for show"—that would be frivolous and suit no purpose. Aprons were meant to keep you clean, not make you pretty. So, in the perspective of my girlhood, I wonder—what kind of woman wore apron No. 13? Was she elegant? Did she keep her apron in a tissue-lined, lavender-scented drawer, and wear it with silk and lace dresses?

My mother kept her mostly faded aprons in the water-heater closet off the kitchen. Ah, they were always nice and warm. This coziness was especially appreciated during long Minnesota winters. My sister Nola and I wore them daily. We wore them well, and we wore them until they were threadbare. Women's work required a sensible apron. Heavens, not one of our four brothers *ever* put on an apron. Men's work on our dairy farm required durable, denim bib overalls—their apron of sorts. Packages of overalls arrived from the Sears Roebuck Company catalog. Nola and I didn't receive packages from Sears Roebuck. Mother never purchased an apron or clothes for us. Why would she do that when she could sew what we needed in minutes from a feed or flour sack? Mother's apron designs covered the bosom, and they all had pockets. We carried handkerchiefs and measuring spoons in them. The aprons were long and gathered at the waist, to provide extra coverage and ease in taking long strides as we went about our work. They protected us from the milk spills while separating milk from cream, flour and sugar spatters while making pies, cookies, and canning peaches. I thought it was silly to wear an apron in the garden like my mother did. She rarely took hers off. On our farm everything had to be practical.

I had a favorite apron. It was patches of wildflowers. I liked the way I could wrap the ties front to back and around again to make a bow in the front instead of the back. Maybe I wanted to be just a little bit frilly after all.

Since I have adopted an apron to which I cannot relate, I must take extra care to respect the maker and the original owner. She may not have worn it to slaughter the hog, pluck the chickens, or separate the cream from the milk. I wonder. Where did she wear it? What kind of woman was she? Was it a gift and kept in the original box, never to be worn? My mother had some of those. So, I can't make any judgments about the owner of No. 13. For perhaps she butchered the hog, then powdered her nose and changed her apron to entertain her lovely friends.

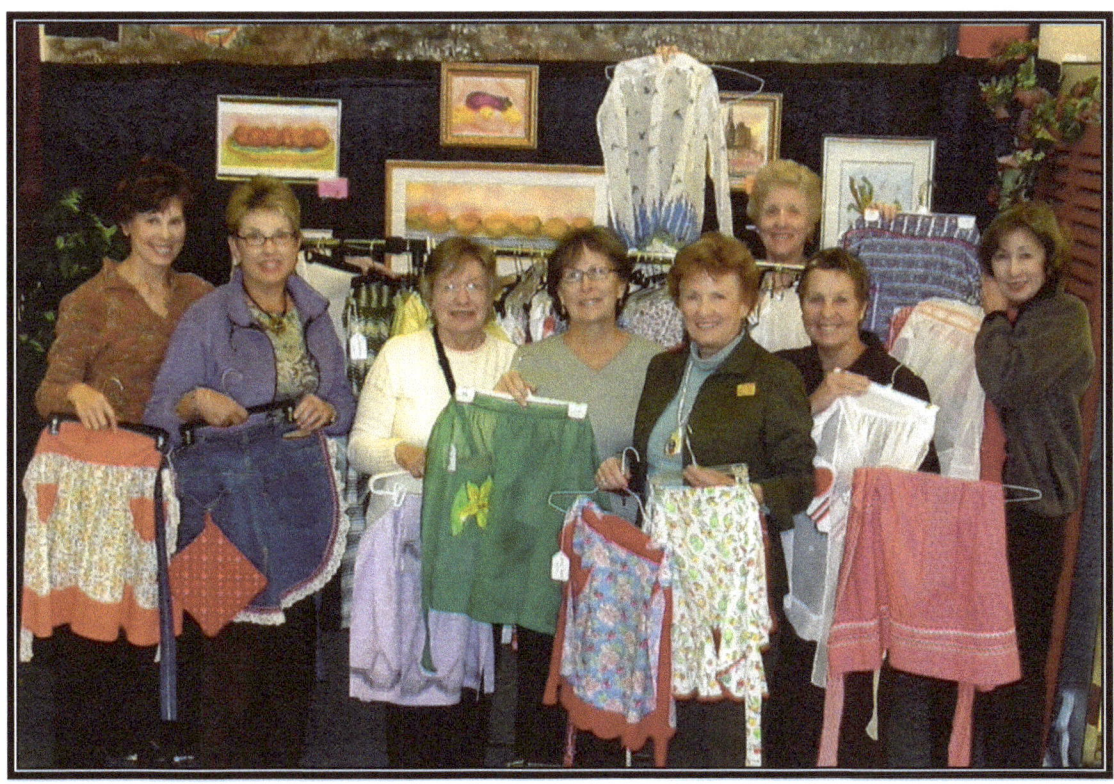

Gotcha Covered contributors meet at Miss Daisy's for lunch and apron time.
(L–R) Marti Mueller Daniel, Ginger T. Manley, Louise Colln, Sue Wilson, Frances Edwards, Poppy Buchanan (in back), Marceleen Alford, Dianne Horton Wood
(Photo courtesy Manley family archives)

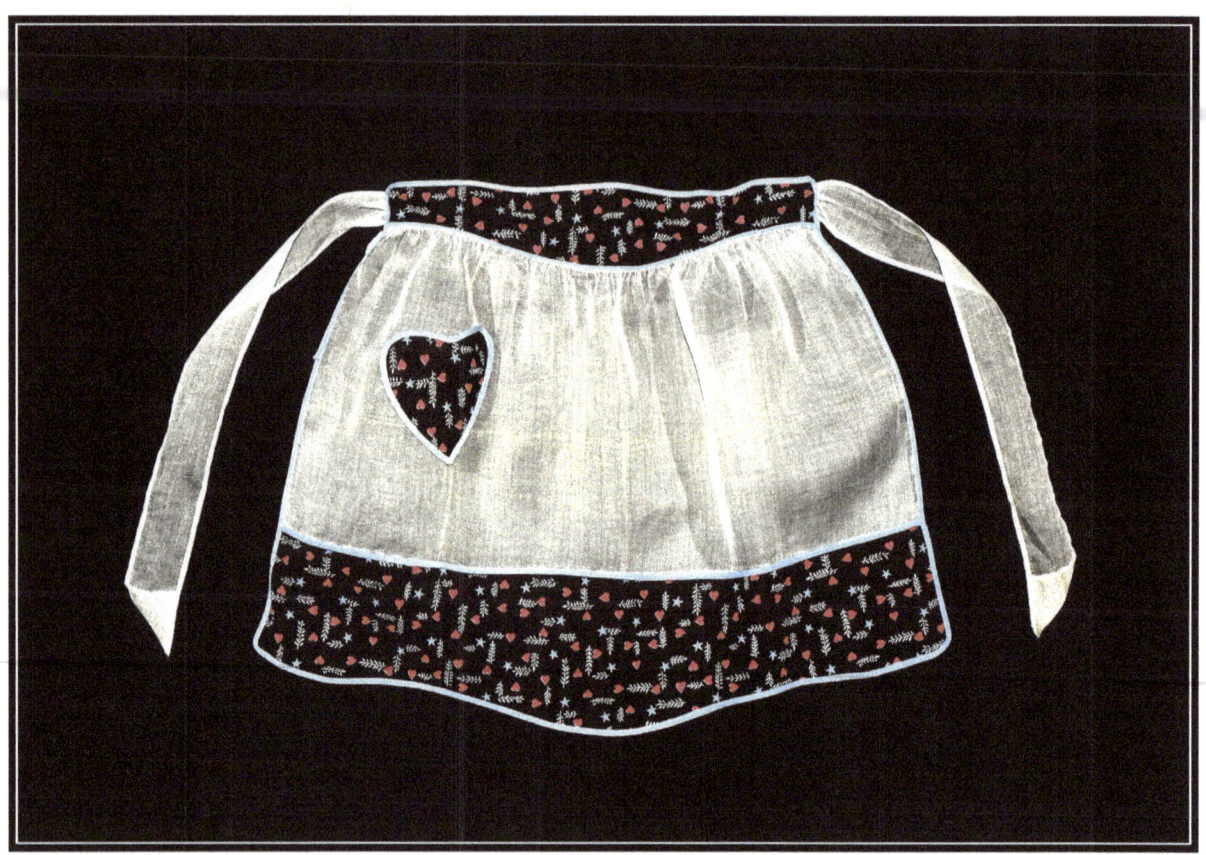

Adopted Summer, 2007 by Maxine Arnold Dalton

The Abandoned Apron

Maxine Arnold Dalton

My apron has been abandoned at least twice. The first time, it was abandoned when its owner moved away from her farm and into a retirement center, where she didn't need to cook anymore. The second time, it was abandoned when the adopter was too busy with other projects to give the apron much thought. Agreeing to accept the gift of the abandoned apron has led me to think about how it was that I, too, came to abandon aprons, and why it is that in my later years I have taken them up again.

Because of the events that occurred in America as my generation graduated from college, the story of abandoned aprons is the story of the second coming of age of my generation. After my widowed grandmother, Louise Elizabeth Anna Freund, gave up housekeeping, she moved amongst the homes of her three daughters and lived part of each year with our family. Like many women of her time, she always wore a bib-styled apron that slipped over her neck and tied at the waist. She wore her apron when she made biscuits, quilted, crocheted, made rag rugs, and surreptitiously helped me with my ironing when the basket in my room was overflowing.

My mother also wore an apron. I have no memory of a particular one, except that hers were also bib-style. She sewed and cooked, and drove me and my brothers and sister to music lessons, Little League games, and friend's houses. Since she had grown up in Nashville, when it was time for me to go to college, she pushed me toward a bachelor's degree in nursing at Vanderbilt. My mother had not been able to attend college because her mother was a widow and there was no money.

My formative years were the 1950s, and so I never thought to protest that I was not allowed to wear slacks or shorts on campus. If I was going to the tennis courts, I was required to wear a raincoat over my shorts or slacks. After graduation in 1962, I joined the parade and married. I had babies and I, too, wore an apron. In fact, I am almost positive that one of my wedding presents was a little organdy apron. It had to be ironed. In fact, it was very much like my adopted apron, but it had embroidery rather than patterned trim and appliqué.

My adopted apron looks like it could have been handmade from one of those patterns that ran in the Women's section of the newspaper. Like the adopted apron, my wedding present apron was too small to provide any protection from spills and splatters, and was more symbolic than functional. What was the point of these pretty little aprons? Did we wear them with heels when we served dinner to our guests or lunch to the bridge group?

I do remember another handmade apron. I made it in home economics class. It was white, made of some kind of regulation muslin or flour sacking, and the purpose of making it was to learn how to hand stitch the binding around the apron. As I recall, the binding was blue. We used this apron to protect our clothing during the cooking unit of the home economics class. Need I say that only girls took home economics? Boys took shop. What happened to this apron after home economics class has faded from my memory. I guess it was abandoned, but it was very practical and had a bib.

As a young mother, I wore an apron and gave little dinner parties. I joined the League of Women Voters, and wore gloves and a hat to church. I watched the world around me—the sit-ins, the Beatles, the assassinations, the war, the sex, drugs, and rock 'n' roll, and the Women's Movement. My marriage fell apart and I became a single mother. As a full-blown feminist coming to terms with the first thirty years of my life, I gave up my aprons and I gave up ironing. It was a hard time but it was also glorious, like being young for the first time.

I joined countless consciousness-raising groups and support groups. One was called The Wednesday Evening Support and Hit Group, which still meets from time to time. One was called Lust for Theory: a Marxist Feminist study group—in which we practiced arguing ideas without getting angry at our antagonist or bursting into tears. My friends and I—a number of whom had been nurses—returned to school for PhDs, and degrees in law and medicine, and still we wore no aprons. I worked very hard to attend school and support my children. Such heady days they were.

The members of the Wednesday Evening Support and Hit Group had T-shirts made, emblazoned with the slogan "No Time for Cookies," to show how liberated we were. In truth, being children of the '50s, we felt some guilt that our children had to take store-bought cookies to school functions because we were all too busy to cook. But we told ourselves otherwise.

And so, the years have gone by and now I am retired. I spend a lot more time cooking than in those years of graduate school when I was mothering, working, and the like. My daughter brought me to tears recently, thanking me for having served dinner every night at the table as she was growing up—meat, a starch, and a vegetable. No doubt the influence of the home economics class.

And now, I bake and cook and garden. I am grateful for all of the women in my life that wore aprons and taught me how to quilt, and sew, and think for myself. I am grateful for the years of following the rules and doing what was expected, because the contrast with the years that followed without an apron—and breaking the rules—are sharp and clear, and make me smile. I am grateful to be the age that I am, able to go and be and do as I please, surrounded by children, grandchildren, wonderful friends, and a dear husband.

But when I lean against the sink or the counter to wash dishes, chop vegetables, roll out crusts, etc., I keep ruining my shirts with stains right above the belly button. I remember that I once gave my husband an apron to wear when he cooks outside. So, I have taken back the gift, his red apron, and when I want to be sure not to get spots on the front of my shirt, I wear my red apron. It has a bib. It does not need to be ironed.

Welcome, abandoned apron, into my life. I have told you my story. I wish that you could tell me yours. But now I am trying to remember—when I was with my granddaughter making chocolate chip cookies a few weeks back, did either of us wear an apron? I wonder if I should buy her one?

SERVICE LEGACIES

Gotcha Covered: A Legacy of Service and Protection

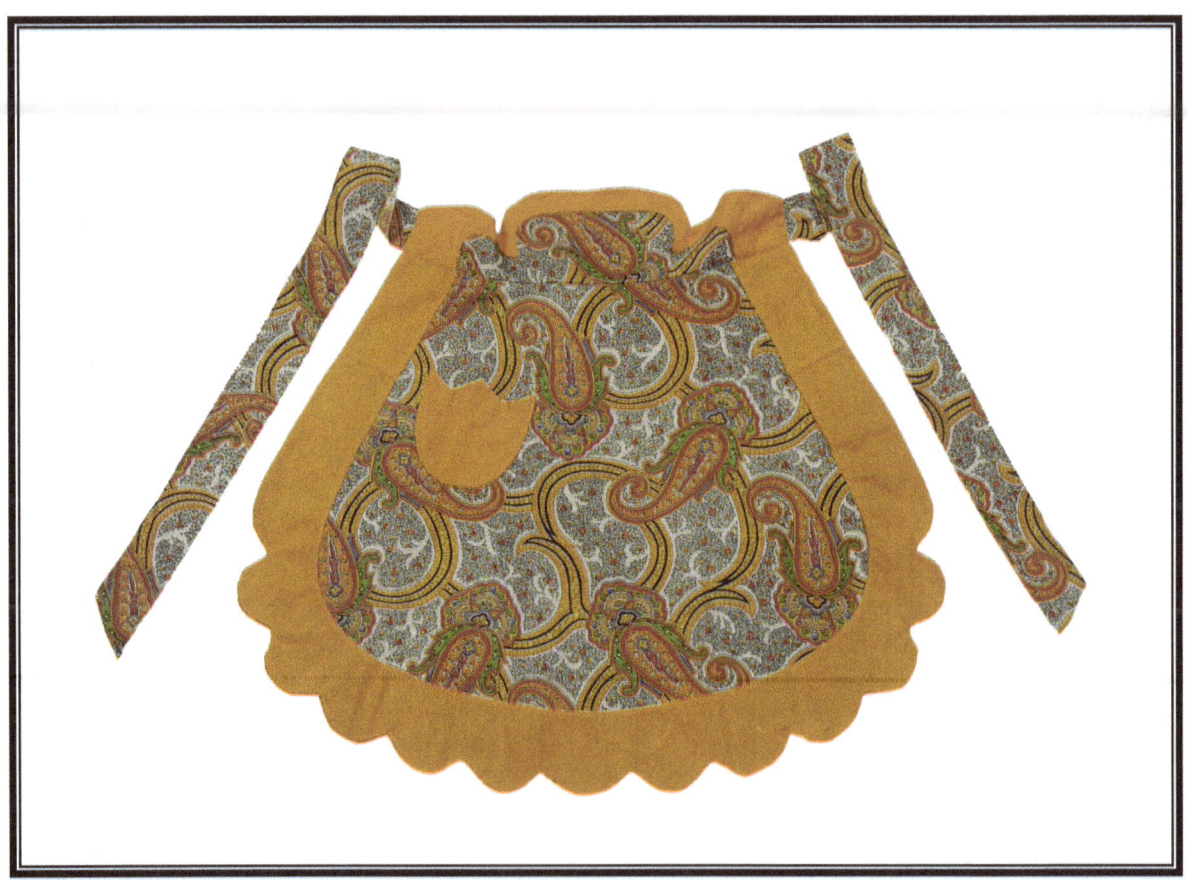

Adopted March 24, 2007 by Krista Koleas

An Apron of Service

Krista Koleas

Dear beloved friends,

You, who have made my life so rich and so meaningful.

I have recently received an apron of many vibrant and lovely colors, all arranged in a joyful pattern. At first glance, all one might see is something beautiful. Looking deeper, its purpose and reason for being slowly emerges. Aprons signify service. They were designed to be worn by those who are giving to others, like a mother cooking for her family, an artist pouring himself into a masterpiece, or a nurse bathing her patient. All are varied expressions of submissiveness, generosity, and sharing. The colors in this apron are a simple expression of all the unique ways in which we may give of ourselves, extend ourselves, and enter into the lives of others. I hope that this adopted apron will remind me to always be willing to serve others, in any way in which I am capable.

To those who have served me . . . my apron is you.

You have been patient when I was not myself.

You have been gentle when I was messy.

You have been present when you could have run.

You have listened to me.

You have given me time when you had little to spare.

You have shown me grace when I got it all wrong.

You have given me courage when fear controlled me.

You have forgiven me.

You have been consistent when my mind changed daily.

You have guided me when I did not have eyes to see.

You have been my strength when I was too weak to try harder.

You have loved me.

Just as Jesus took up His apron to serve His disciples by washing their feet, so have you washed mine numerous times. In all your ways with me, I have seen Jesus. I hope I will never forget what a privilege it is to serve you, and that I will wear my apron with the same compassion and selflessness that you have worn yours.

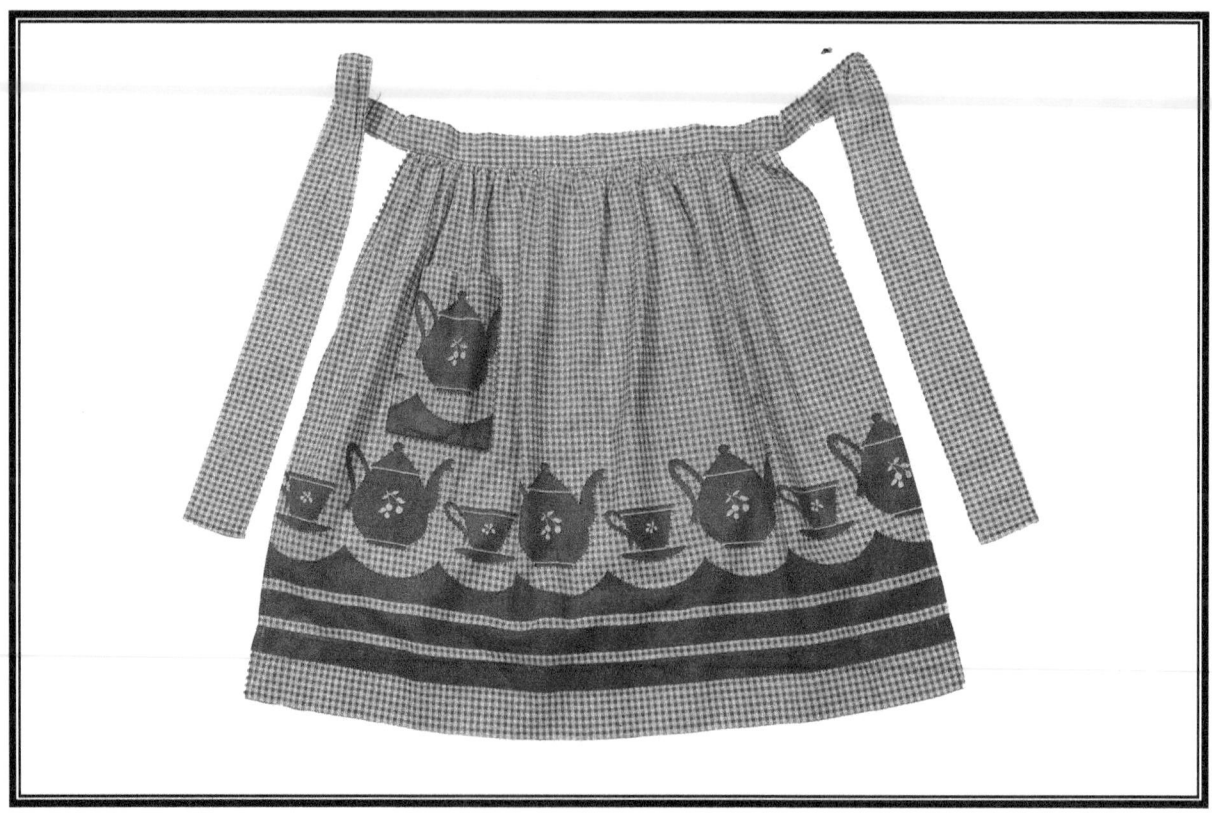

Adopted December 4, 2006 by Margaret Kuehnle Fulton

The Word: Hospitality

Margaret Kuehnle Fulton

In the Bible there's a story that's perplexed me now and then.
    About Jesus and two sisters and what happened way back when.
    Martha's apron fluttered smartly, as she fretted and she fussed.
    Showing kindness to all guests was her divine and sacred trust.
She stayed busy in the kitchen trying best to serve her Lord.
    Mary sat at Jesus' feet, absorbing every spoken word.
The part of me resembling Mary would've rather been with her.
    But the me that's more like Martha would've thought, "I have to serve."
Someone had to cook and wait upon, she'd learned through years of toil.
    So her sister's role seemed selfish; her own rooted in her soul.
I understand poor Martha and can very well relate.
    It was a big occasion—she was burdened by her state.
My nature is to organize, making sure the job gets done.
    But I would've been unsettled—felt I'd missed out on the fun.
Martha asked the Lord for help, crying, "Jesus, please do tell
    My sister Mary to come in here and help me for a spell."
His response, so unexpected, left her worries nigh unheeded,
    "Martha, all your troubled feelings are surely not here needed."
His next words came, oh, so gently, but they gave her quite a start,
    "For herself, your sister Mary has but chosen the best part."
I have asked the Lord so many times, "How can I find this bliss?"
    At long last and with great gratitude, I know what's been amiss.
It's good to be hospitable and kind, of that we're sure.
    But, first grasp His love and truth—the One that does endure.
Take the time to learn from Jesus—let Him fill you to the brim.
    With his strength and wisdom guiding, you can never fail with Him.
When you choose the best part first, serving others comes to be.
    Thank the Lord He cares so much to help the Martha that is me!

The blue and white gingham apron with the border of teapots, cups, and saucers conjured thoughts for Margaret of serving company and showing hospitality.

GOTCHA COVERED: A LEGACY OF SERVICE AND PROTECTION

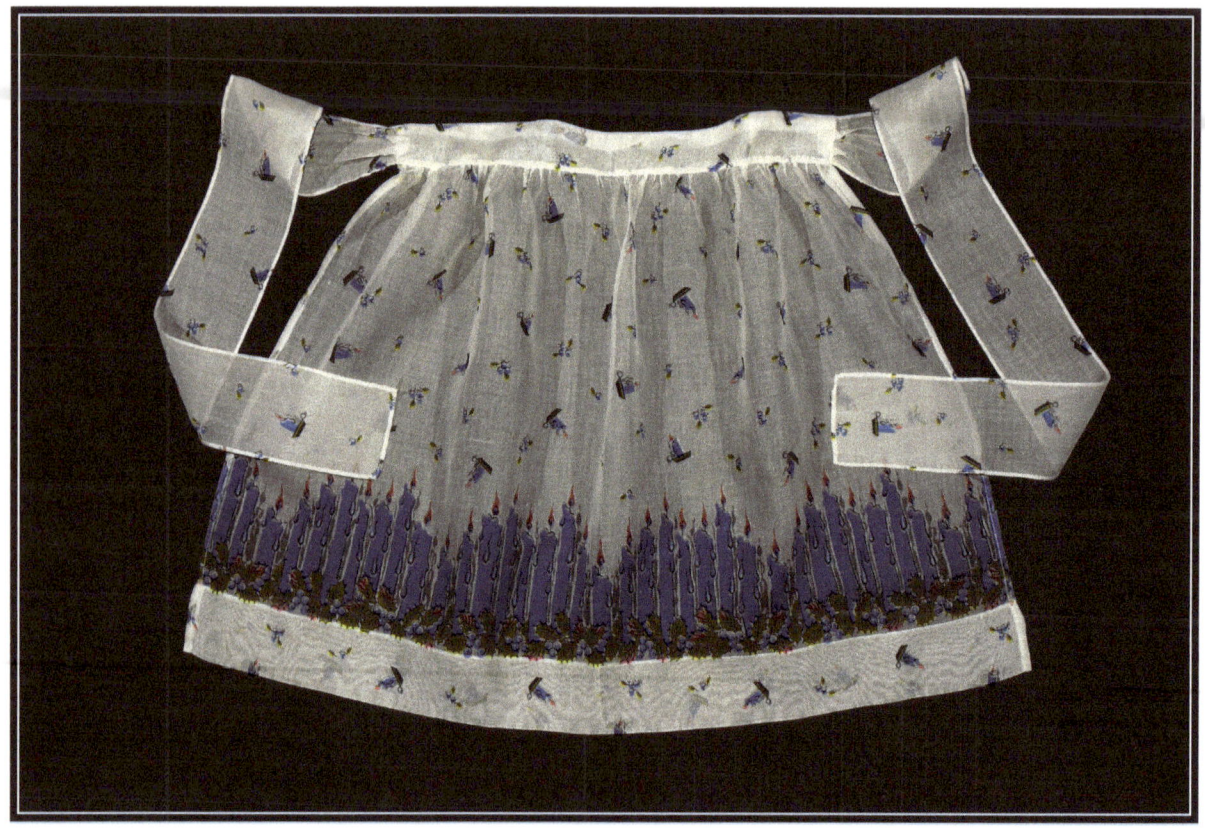

Adopted March 8, 2007 by Poppy Pickering Buchanan

Celebrate Life

Poppy Pickering Buchanan

Join with family, friends, and even strangers to respond with enthusiasm to every occasion.
Prepare food, decorate, dress up, and get ready to receive guests.
Mother, with an apron tied around her waist, meant she was ready to serve her guests.
It announced that dinner was ready.
She had finished setting the table and preparing the food, and she could enjoy being at her party.
The three daughters would clear the table and do the dishes.
Family celebrations to me were times of laughter and happy conversation.
It was as if no unpleasantness would be allowed at the table.
Maybe we should wear an apron to prepare every meal, and sit down and enjoy without unpleasantness the joy of being in this life together.

PART THREE: *Aprons as Symbols of Comfort*

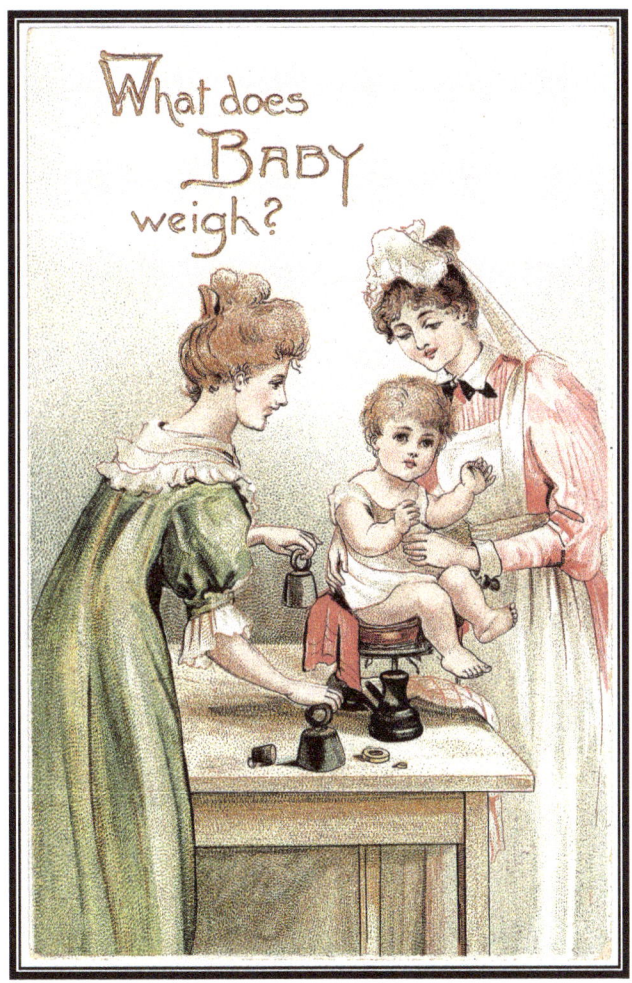

© Zwerdling Nursing Archives, used with permission.

Aprons as Symbols of Comfort

Ginger T. Manley

There is comfort food and comfort clothing. Mashed potatoes and gravy, meatloaf, and apple crisp are comfort foods we can all relate to. Aprons, in my mind, constitute the notion of "comfort clothes." I always feel perfectly comfortable in an apron—like an anachronism, but perfectly comfortable.

Marcy Goldman, www.betterbaking.com

For several years women have been sending their friends, via the Internet, the following story based on the poem, *Grandma's Apron*, written by Tina Trivett (2007) as a tribute to her grandmother.

The principal use of Grandma's apron was to protect the dress underneath, but along with that, it served as a potholder for removing hot pans from the oven. It was wonderful for drying children's tears, and on occasion was even used for cleaning out dirty ears. From the chicken coop, the apron was used for carrying eggs, fussy chicks, and sometimes half-hatched eggs to be finished in the warming oven. When company came, those aprons were ideal hiding places for shy kids. And when the weather was cold, grandma wrapped it around her arms. Those big old aprons wiped many a perspiring brow bent over the hot wood stove. Chips and kindling wood were brought into the kitchen in that apron. From the garden, it carried all sorts of vegetables. After the peas had been shelled, it carried out the hulls. In the fall the apron was used to bring in apples that had fallen from the trees. When unexpected company drove up the road, it was surprising how much furniture that old apron could dust in a matter of seconds. When dinner was ready, Grandma walked out onto the porch, waved her apron, and the men knew it was time to come in from the fields to dinner. It will be a long time before someone invents something that will replace the "old-time apron" that served so many purposes. (Grandma's Apron)

Somewhere along the transmission line, a woman (probably) added:

Remember, Grandma used to set her hot baked apple pies on the windowsill to cool. Her granddaughters set theirs on the kitchen counter to thaw.

The word *apron* evolved from the old French word *nappe*, meaning "tablecloth," and then its derivative, *naperon*, meaning "table napkin." In English, this evolution became *napron* in the 1400s, then by the late 1600s, the word had become *apron*, or in old English, *aprone*. Before paper was widely available for mapmaking, maps were drawn on cloth, sometimes on the same cloth which had been used in the service of dinner, either a cloth napkin or cloth apron. Aprons, either serving as literal map material or as protection for clothing, have defined territory for both genders for thousands of years.

Utility aprons started out as pieces of cloth or leather worn by men in their places of work. In this particular section of the anthology, all the apron memories are associated with modern utility aprons worn by women in their domestic territories—usually the kitchen, but sometimes the laundry room or garden.

More than half the contributors to this anthology were inspired to write lovingly of warm and happy memories, of kitchens and homes tended by mothers, grandmothers, aunts, and housemaids who wore aprons. Aprons, as comfort clothes worn in these spaces, trigger powerful emotions of love, sadness, or surprise. Reading these pieces is like a walk backwards into less trying, more secure times. Whether the apron serves as a vehicle that transports us into the kitchen of our memory or the lap of a loved one, we eagerly go there seeking comfort and nurturing.

Kitchen Legacies

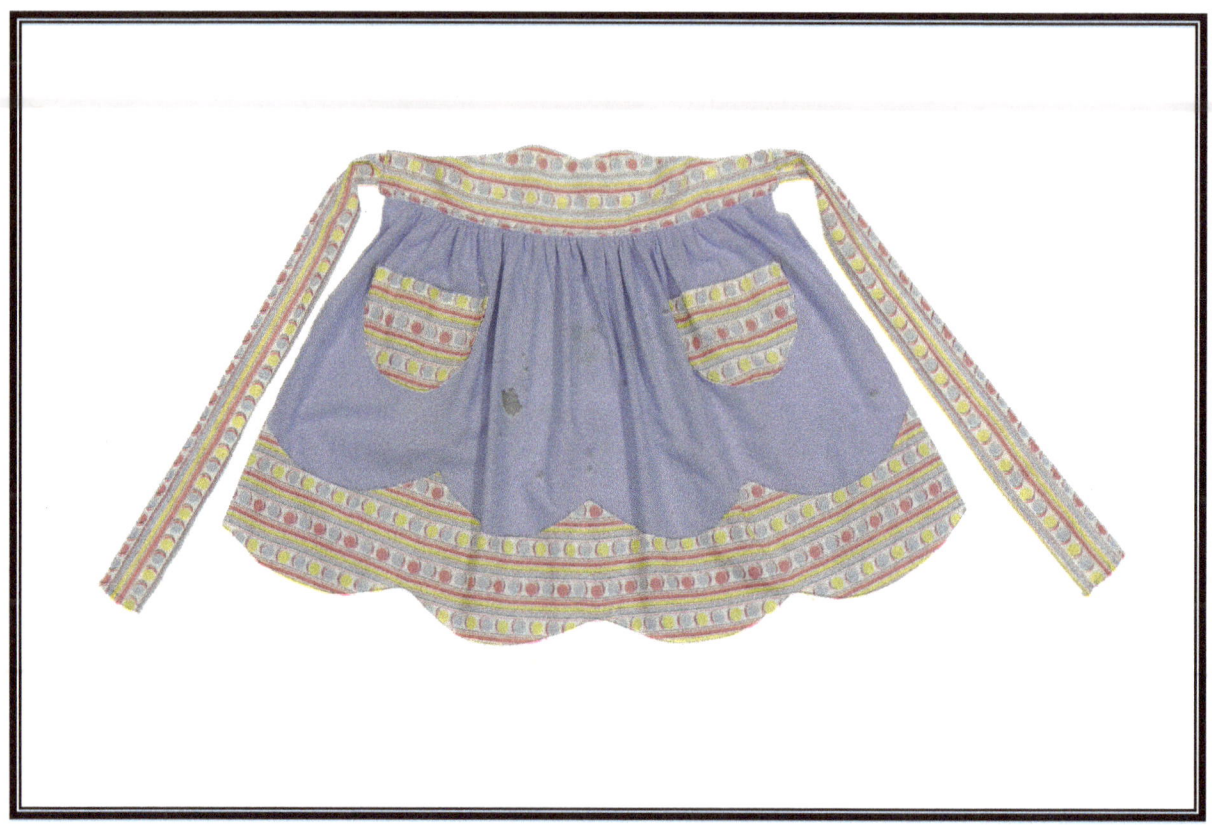

Adopted November 10, 2006 by Sally Reinhart Crowe

GOTCHA COVERED: A LEGACY OF SERVICE AND PROTECTION

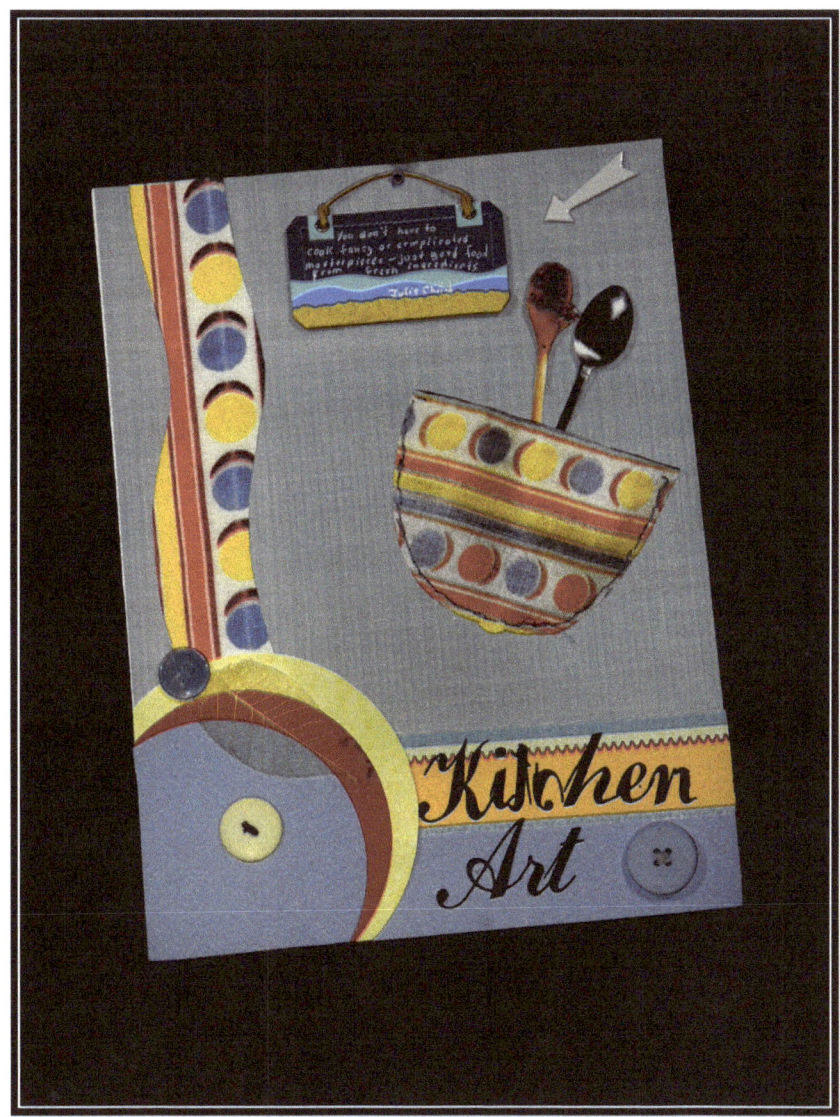

Sally Crowe was inspired by her adopted apron to create this paper collage using photo-reproductions of the original apron fabric.

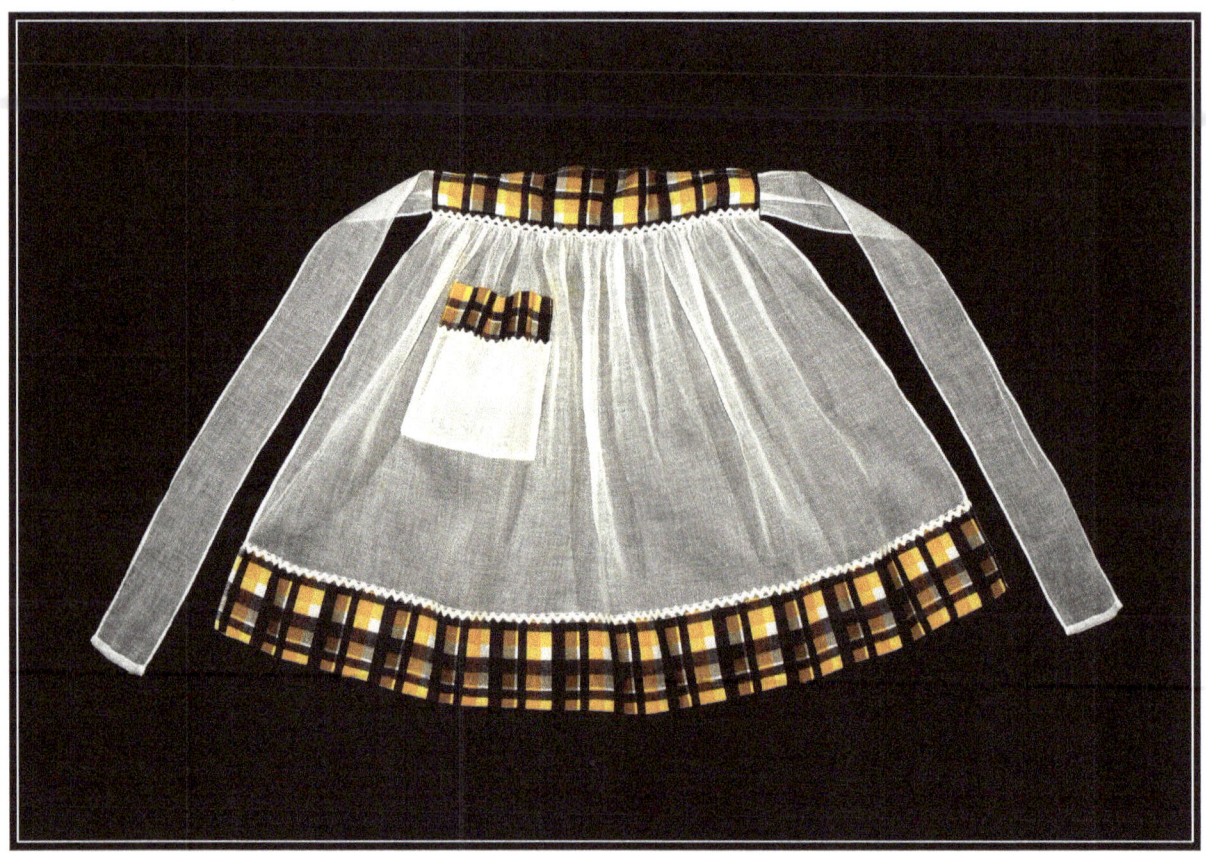

Adopted April 7, 2007 by Sharron Stewart Burch

Little Apron

Sharron Stewart Burch

I'm a little apron
    starched and white.
      Just put me on and
    you'll see the light.
Grab a measuring cup
    I'll help you bake.
We'll mix the batter up
      for your birthday cake!

This apron was inadvertently adopted by two separate contributors. Two very different pieces were inspired by the apron.

GOTCHA COVERED: A LEGACY OF SERVICE AND PROTECTION

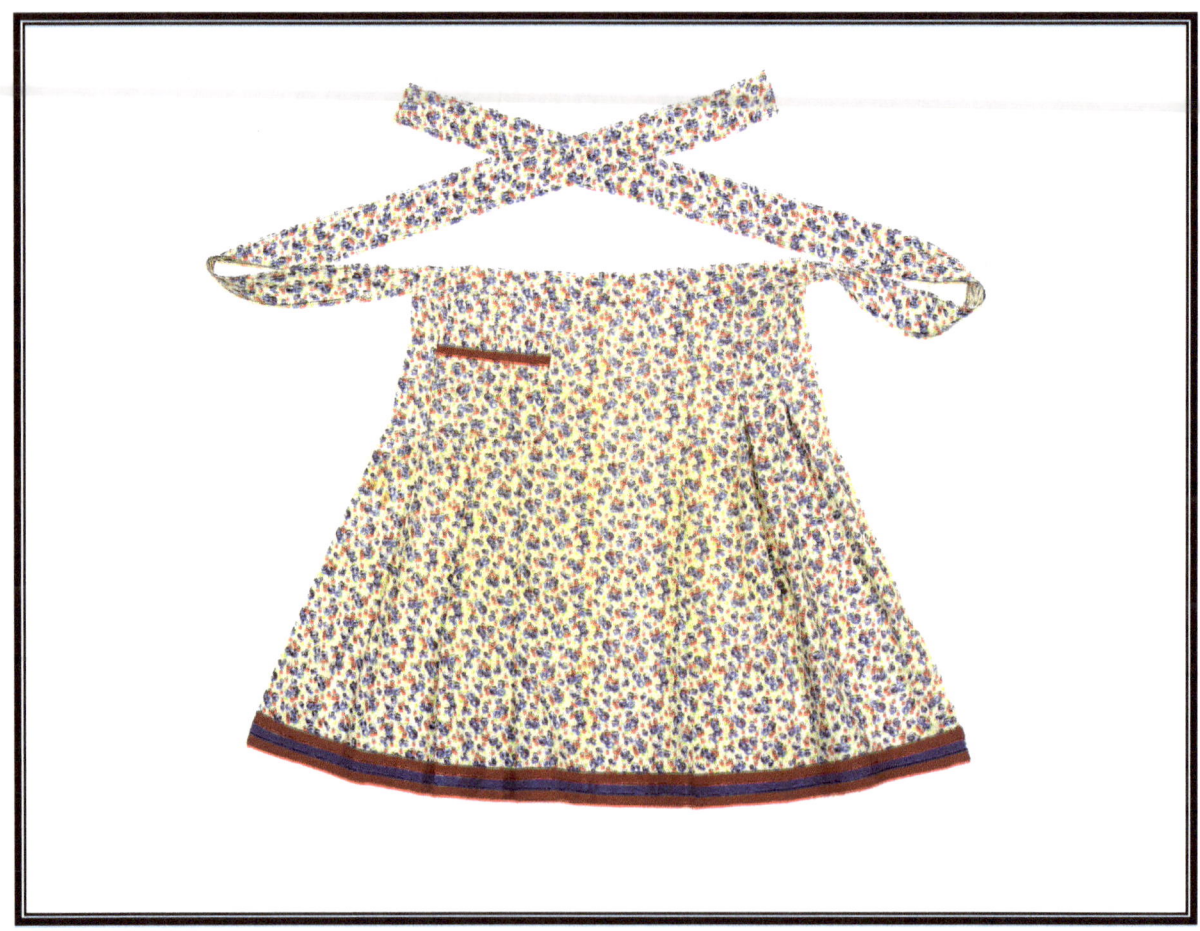

Adopted January 31, 2007 by Linda Schlesinger Mabry

Look for Us in the Kitchen

Linda Schlesinger Mabry

I hope there's a kitchen in heaven. My loved ones know to look for me there. In fact, I expect to go to heaven straight from my own kitchen, leaving behind a freezer full of food and, less likely, clean dishes. I come from a long line of enthusiastic cooks and have persistent memories of family kitchens where I learned about life and the value of family members who care about each other.

On my father's side of the family, Great-Grandma Crawford made sweet wine from Muscadine grapes and stored it in crocks down in her Tennessee basement. Her son, Henry, was allowed to taste it, but her daughters were not. Once, finding a batch of this medicinal potion, thickened and dark with age, my dad and his brother got the dog drunk. Whether or not the boys tasted it themselves remains a secret.

Other family members had their specialties. Great-Grandma Schlesinger had a way with fresh spinach. Plain Grandma, my paternal grandmother, had a way with hot fudge sauce, which was always in the blue pitcher when we visited. It thickened just right when poured over vanilla ice cream. ("Plain Grandma" was my way of differentiating the grandmother with the same last name as mine [Schlesinger] from the one with a different last name.) Plain Grandpa loved salty country ham and made his redeye gravy with coffee in it. On special occasions, he made taffy, which the kids got to pull with him. He let us dig potatoes, pick cukes for bread & butter pickles, and gather huge blackberries from the fencerow along his garden. There, he taught us ditties like:

Pie, pie 'tater pie
p - i - e - e - i - p - pie.
E for, *i* for, eat a piece of pie, for
we just love that 'tater pie.

When we wondered how anyone could eat a pie made of vegetables, Grandma made such a pie for us. I never see a sweet potato pie without the urge to burst into song.

On Mother's side of the family, Grandma Stoughton's German doughnuts, fragrant with mace, were an unusual treat. For special occasions, she made a sherry pudding and brought in bowls of her beautiful roses for the table. To this day, I prefer my grapefruit with salt and my cantaloupe with pepper, like they season them in Texas. The Stoughtons lived in Dallas and ran their neighborhood grocery store next door. When we visited, they let me mind the store. Grandpa was a wiry, hardworking man with the softest of hearts. It was his practice to run a tab for people who did not have the money for their purchases. He always let us fill a bag with candy and Devil Dogs from their store to take on the long drive home. Maybe I can attribute to him my attraction to candy bars.

During the early fifties in Houston, Texas, my family had a modern, chrome and red Formica dinette set, with matching chairs that grabbed the skin on our skinny, bare legs. In the sticky climate (no air conditioning), the breeze from the black oscillating fan accompanied meals for much of the year.

A finicky eater through all of childhood, I must have been a disappointment at the table. My sister and I drank so much chocolate milk that the non-flavored version was referred to as "white milk." There was only whole milk at the time; my grandmother referred to it as "homogenized milk." She grew up with fresh milk, which had the cream risen to the top and needed shaking to mix before drinking. One of us spilled our milk at almost every meal. Was it rambunctious girls or unstable glasses? We lived the fifties' ideal of family togetherness, and supper together was a ritual. It was there that we eventually learned table manners, and now we rarely spill our milk.

We saw the dawn of a new age in food. Chemists were dreaming up new food products, advertised to people of modest means and eagerly adopted by the public. Fresh foods were replaced by convenience foods, with long lists of ingredients and additives. I remember when Oreos and sugared breakfast cereals were new. Frozen TV dinners became available, but my family never ate them, preferring home-cooked meals. I find it difficult to forget Mama's standbys in those days, the creamed chipped beef on toast, fish sticks, meat loaf, hash (a name for beef stew), wedges of iceberg lettuce with bottled French dressing, and canned green beans cooked in a pressure cooker. As we dawdled reluctantly over each bite, we kids were frequently admonished to appreciate what we had, since there were starving children in China. With no clear idea of the whereabouts of those children, I was more than willing to send them my food. But her homemade pies and cakes were THE BEST, and that motivated me to clean my plate.

We carried our lunches to Will Rogers Elementary School—sandwiches on soft, white bread with the crusts cut off to eliminate any texture, and always cut in triangles and wrapped in wax paper. After lunch in the school cafeteria, we had regular drills, getting under our desks or lining up in the hall with our hands protecting our little necks from nuclear bombs and tornadoes.

After-school snacks were an enticement to share our day's experience. It was at snack time that we first heard a favorite family tale. "Mama, tell us about the time you poured soup in my hair," I would plead. I'm told I poured my cool, congealed Campbell's tomato soup in my innocent and unsuspecting sister's hair. Shocking us all, my exasperated mother poured soup in my hair to teach me a lesson, only to create a grand mess for herself.

Moments like these have reassured me that maybe I could be a good parent without losing myself. We don't have to behave perfectly all the time, but there are consequences. The soup story was my earliest indication that Mama was a real person, not just my mother. I got the occasional, uneasy feeling that she wondered, who *are* these little girls and when is their real mother going to come and get them? When she said, "You are driving me to the loony bin and you'll have to visit me there," that was our clue to back off for a while. Thank goodness she stayed to see that we were "raised right." She may argue that she was not the perfect mother, but she is the perfect mother for me. I know there is always a place for me and mine at her table, where each of us feels loved from every direction and buffered from the ugly or frightening parts of life.

In the fifties, moms wore aprons in the kitchen, while dads got dressed, had breakfast and coffee, and went off in the family's one car to work in the world beyond the neighborhood. Unable to comprehend or explain what a chemical engineer did at a paint and varnish company, I told people my daddy painted houses. He did paint ours, with full family participation. I lived for the day I could be the one on the ladder. In an extension of his work, he was always "cooking up" some product for us to use at home—cleaners, sunscreen, insect repellent, shampoo, colored concrete for our driveway, and more. These no-name-brand substitutes for commercial products were slow to gain family acceptance. He was experimental, too, when he cooked food. I remember the potatoes, dropped into boiling resin, while he grilled on the cooker he made from a fifty-gallon paint drum. Considering recipes as formulas to be refined and tested was an engineer's approach to food, and not a bad legacy. His experimentation left us open to change, when the food revolution of the early seventies freed us from the reliance on convenience foods and led us back to "from scratch" cooking.

Through the changes of the years, the family has gathered to share food. We are how we eat, and who's at the table is more important than what is on it. Still, what's on the table draws my family there. Look for us in the kitchen.

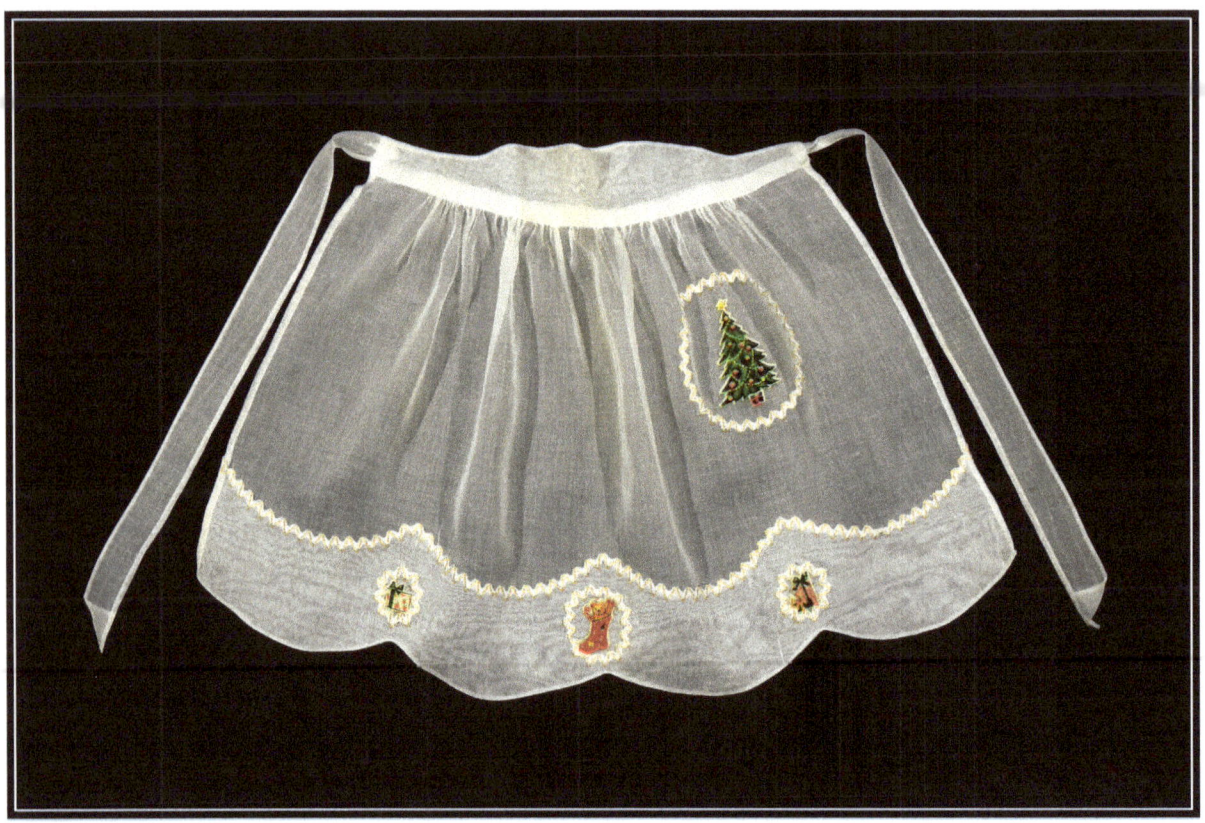

Adopted March 29, 2007 by Donna Maddox

The Apron

Donna Maddox

The last "Away in a Manger" had been sung and we had exchanged Christmas cards. There was much excitement in the classroom on our last day before Christmas vacation. As we began leaving the classroom, we gave each other hugs and best wishes for a "Merry Christmas." Since I would be leaving for Petersburg the next day, I received a few extra hugs.

After school, I began packing the gifts Auntie and I had wrapped for me to take to Mama. There were also some that she and others had wrapped for me. Early the next morning, I boarded the Norfolk & Western super train, *The Powhatan Arrow*, named after Pocahontas' father. Six hours later I arrived in Petersburg, VA, and as always when I made this trip, I saw Mama waiting for me in front of the station. I rushed from the train and into her arms for hugs and kisses. Before we headed home, she always took me into the station for a bowl of their excellent Brunswick stew. She watched as I ate.

Once home, Mama helped me unpack and set our gifts aside. In the morning we would shop for our tree and decorate it the next night. In the meantime, we made out a grocery list and went shopping for our Christmas delights and "makings" for our Christmas dinner. Mama always liked for me to go with her to the grocery store because she wanted to get the things I most liked to eat. Because I was "home" and with her only for Christmases and summers, she never knew what my favorite foods might be.

With groceries unloaded, tree decorated, and gifts placed around the tree, Mama was ready to don her Christmas apron and to begin to prepare for our holiday feasts. Looking back, I can almost smell the turkey baking in the oven and see her tasting the gravy with a wooden spoon. She would place the pies on the windowsill to cool and brew the sweet tea to perfection.

Each year was the same, more or less, with Mama donning her apron and cooking for the holidays. Then came sharing our treats with family and friends. There were always open houses to attend, and beautifully decorated churches to attend to hear Christmas carols and praise and worship for our Savior on His birthday.

Now, years have passed since those wonderful days in Petersburg with Mama. But when the festive spirit of Christmas approaches, I reach in the bottom drawer of my chest for Mama's Christmas apron and hug it close. It is quite old now—more than sixty years old. It is faded and wonderfully worn with age. But, oh, the memories it holds for me. Mama's love seems to pour from it when I tie the strings around my waist and head for the kitchen.

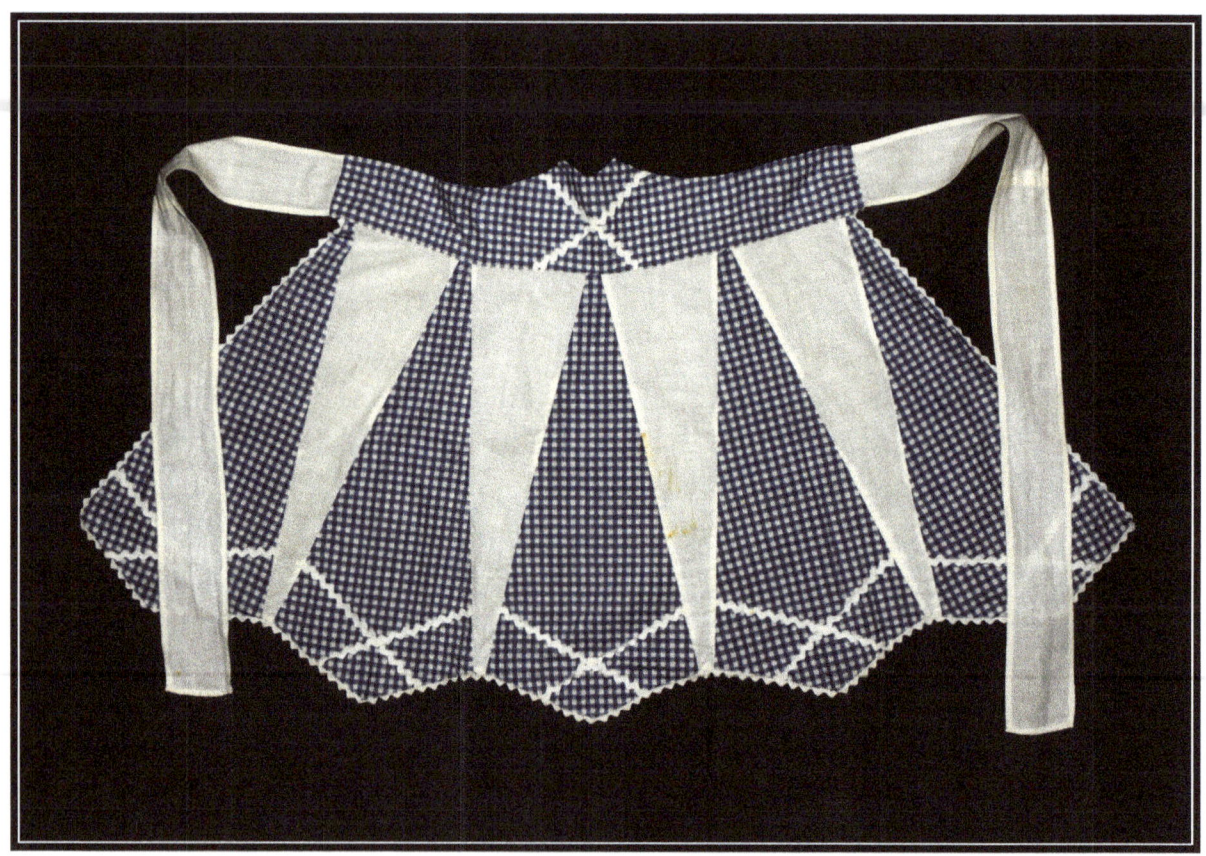

Adopted October 21, 2006 by Sally Yeagley

Coming of Age One Month Before Thanksgiving

Sally Yeagley

I love the color blue. Red and certain greens are acceptable, but I could live the rest of my life surrounded by the color blue. When my older sister, Elizabeth, called and told me she had invited our entire family to my house for Thanksgiving, I knew that I'd want to have blue close to me for comfort.

Maybe I am a big baby, but this is the first time I'll be entertaining the entire family. Sister must be testing me. I've only been out of college for six months, and married for five. Entertaining a few couples isn't anything like having the entire family at once. I felt so confident at college graduation, but now as a new wife in a new home, I am a little nervous about my new responsibilities.

Bill and I loved this house the minute we drove in the driveway. Glen, our real estate agent, showed us several houses. When we drove up to this two-story colonial wonder, painted the softest wrap-me-in-a-blanket blue, just on the edge of town, I melted. The yard is the size of two houses, and the gardens are full of lovingly tended flowers. That day, my eyes were drawn to the bluebells and to the striking periwinkle hydrangeas. We knew this was the place for Bill and me to raise our family and to entertain. My family had been holding their breath, waiting to see where we decided to live, probably measuring the footage behind my back to see if our extended family of twenty-two could sit, eat, and play for the holidays.

Looks like the place measured up, for everyone is coming for Thanksgiving.

Elizabeth is a natural, confident hostess, the grand organizer who knows just the right people to call for every occasion. She always seems to come out on top. Her husband, George, teaches math at the university. She confided in me that they could not afford much more than their little bungalow on a teacher's salary. Their bungalow is sweet, but there just isn't enough room for our entire family.

So here I am, one month before Thanksgiving, in my wonderful ten-year-old—but new to me—blue house, on the edge of town, sitting at the kitchen table looking at my chrysanthemums in the garden, wondering how to cook a turkey. I have tried casseroles and a small ham, but for this occasion, a turkey the size of a small shrub is to be the star of the show. There will be no room for an under-cooked or charred bird. Thank goodness for the cookbooks we received as wedding presents. Maybe if I can manage the big bird, Mom will make her famous Southern, corn bread dressing.

Mom is such a good cook, but she is getting older. Her back hurts and she can't stand up for long periods of time. It is time for her to pass on her apron.

Oh, her apron. She used to get up in the morning and put on her apron before making coffee. She has a special drawer full of different colored aprons. There is an apron for every occasion. When she is cooking a meal, she usually dons her small half-apron. The pockets are stuffed with extra Kleenex tissue, maybe a throat lozenge, a note or two, even a recipe. It seems to be her walking desk. If she is going to spend the day in the kitchen, canning or cooking, then the full, over-her-shoulders apron comes out of the drawer.

When I was younger, she would come home from her women's church meetings with a fresh, new, handmade apron. The church ladies collected remnants of cloth, maybe from a child's dress or a used skirt, and created an original apron, adding buttons, rickrack, and dainty pockets for dress-up or big wide pockets for everyday. Every apron was a little different, each special in its own way. The churchwomen would exchange aprons. I remember my friend Karen's mom wearing an apron my mother made. It was blue and gold, with gold trim. It made me very proud of my mother.

How am I going to be worthy of wearing an apron? Do I have to be a good cook to wear an apron or do I start with the apron and become a good cook? I guess I will find out Thanksgiving Day.

It's over. Twenty-eight people, to be exact, have left. The dishes are clean and sitting on the dining table; the small Pyrex bowl of leftover turkey on the kitchen table is staring at me, as if asking, "Is that all there is?" Bill is working at his stamp collection. I want to sit and reflect on my first Thanksgiving.

Mr. Johnson, at Johnson's Meat Market, reserved a twenty-two-pound turkey for us. Bill had to help me get it in the oven, and there was no room for anything else. Betty Crocker helped plan the timing and basting, so the turkey was perfect—crisp on the outside and tender-sweet on the inside. Mom made her wonderful dressing, and as always there are no leftovers. Elizabeth had everyone bring a special food. I need to make a note to call Shirley to ask for her sweet potato casserole recipe. That was a yummy treat. The family raved about the house and the table filled with fresh, fall flowers from our garden. Bill was the perfect host. The highballs were just enough to loosen up the crowd, but not enough to send them to bed.

Thanksgiving Day was warm for a change. After dinner we lazily sauntered outside. The children played ball and croquet, while the older family members chatted on the side porch. I am grateful for this day going so well. Elizabeth and Mom took me aside to praise me for a job well done.

Elizabeth knew how nervous I was about having the gathering. I had meant to run to the store for an apron, but it seemed the other tasks were a higher priority. As a surprise, Elizabeth brought me a beautifully wrapped, blue package. When I opened it, there was my apron. Not just a blue apron, not a store-bought apron, but a handmade, white and blue check, gingham apron with white rickrack. The ties are full and white, and the edges are scalloped. This is not a work-around-the-house apron, but a Thanksgiving, dressy apron, handmade by Elizabeth with Mom's help, in my favorite color. It was as if they were passing the torch and adding confidence to my day. It is not a certificate of achievement, but I feel that this apron represents a new phase in my life—the phase of becoming a full-fledged hostess of my own home. I have become a cook, a party organizer, and a grown woman ready to serve her family.

Because of this experience, I have learned that I can tackle any holiday. Bless my sister for my coming-of-age, blue apron.

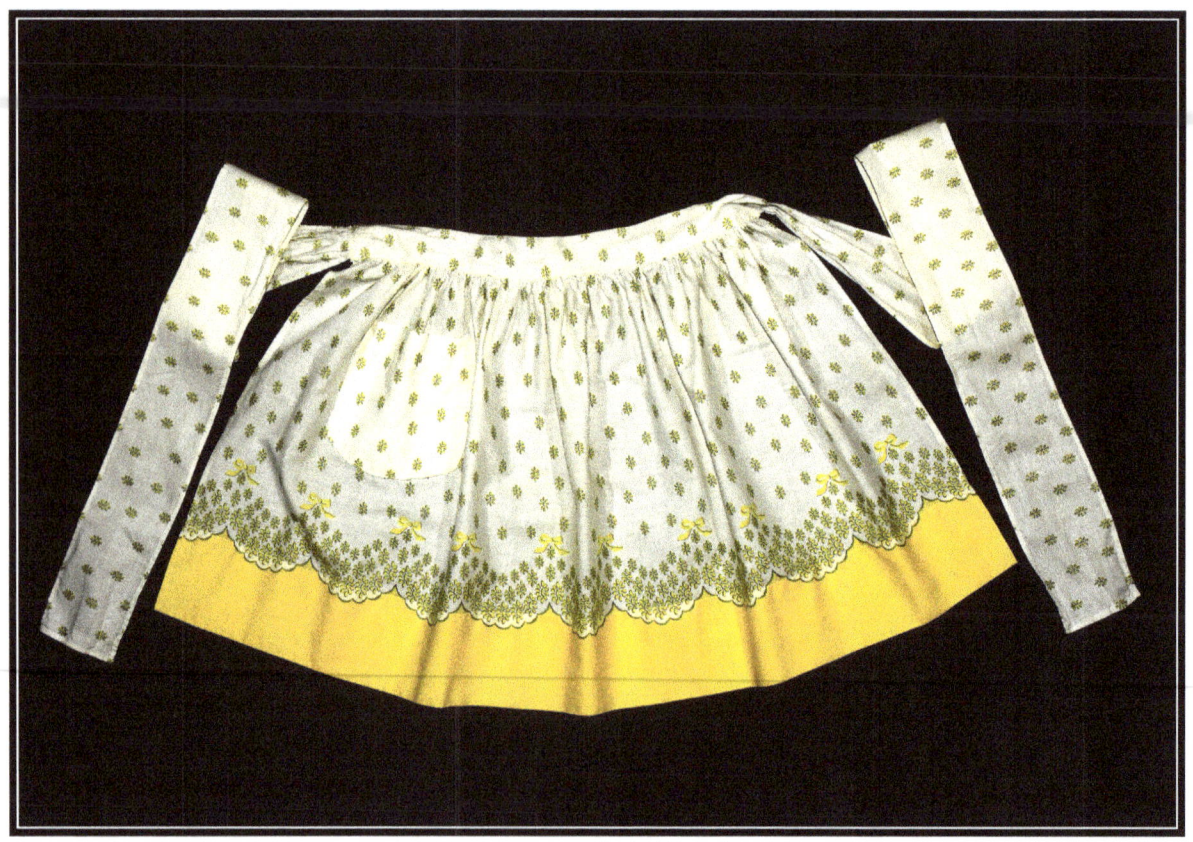

Adopted April 17, 2007 by Lisa Fournace

My Grandma's Kitchen

Lisa Fournace

I can still remember the smells wafting from my Grandma's kitchen filling the whole house, and I can see her apron-clad figure working in the kitchen. She was a truly gifted cook and I believe it was one of her passions.

It was always a treat to go to Grandma's house. I knew when I went there she was going to make sure I was never hungry. She was a true Southern woman, and she definitely knew all about Southern cooking. Her specialty was homemade cakes. She always wore an apron and wiped her hands on it as she worked. I would watch in amazement as she added a dash of this and a pinch of that to create her masterpiece. I anxiously waited for the finished product. I was never encouraged to help her, but I was always allowed to taste-test the final product.

Despite my lack of hands-on experience in her kitchen, I have nevertheless adopted some of her habits in my own kitchen. Like her, I do not measure ingredients. I tuck a towel into my pants to use as my apron. I do not allow people to help me in the kitchen.

My grandmother did not really use recipes. When she passed away, she carried all that knowledge with her. One of my favorite recipes was a lemon cake. I have found a recipe that is the closest to what I remember of hers.

Lemon Cake

1 cup Crisco shortening	2 cups sugar	3 cups flour
4 eggs	1 cup buttermilk	2 tablespoons lemon extract
½ teaspoon baking soda	½ teaspoon baking powder	½ teaspoon salt

Combine all ingredients and mix in a bowl at high speed for 3 minutes. Pour into a greased Bundt pan. Bake at 325° for 1 hour. Keep oven turned on 325°. Loosen edges with knife but do not flip out of pan. Pour the following mixture over the cake.

Lemon Sauce

1 cup powdered sugar	3 tablespoons lemon juice	2 tablespoons orange juice

Mix above sauce ingredients and pour over the cake. Bake in the oven an additional 5 minutes. Let stand 5 minutes and invert over a plate and remove cake from pan.

MOTHERING LEGACIES

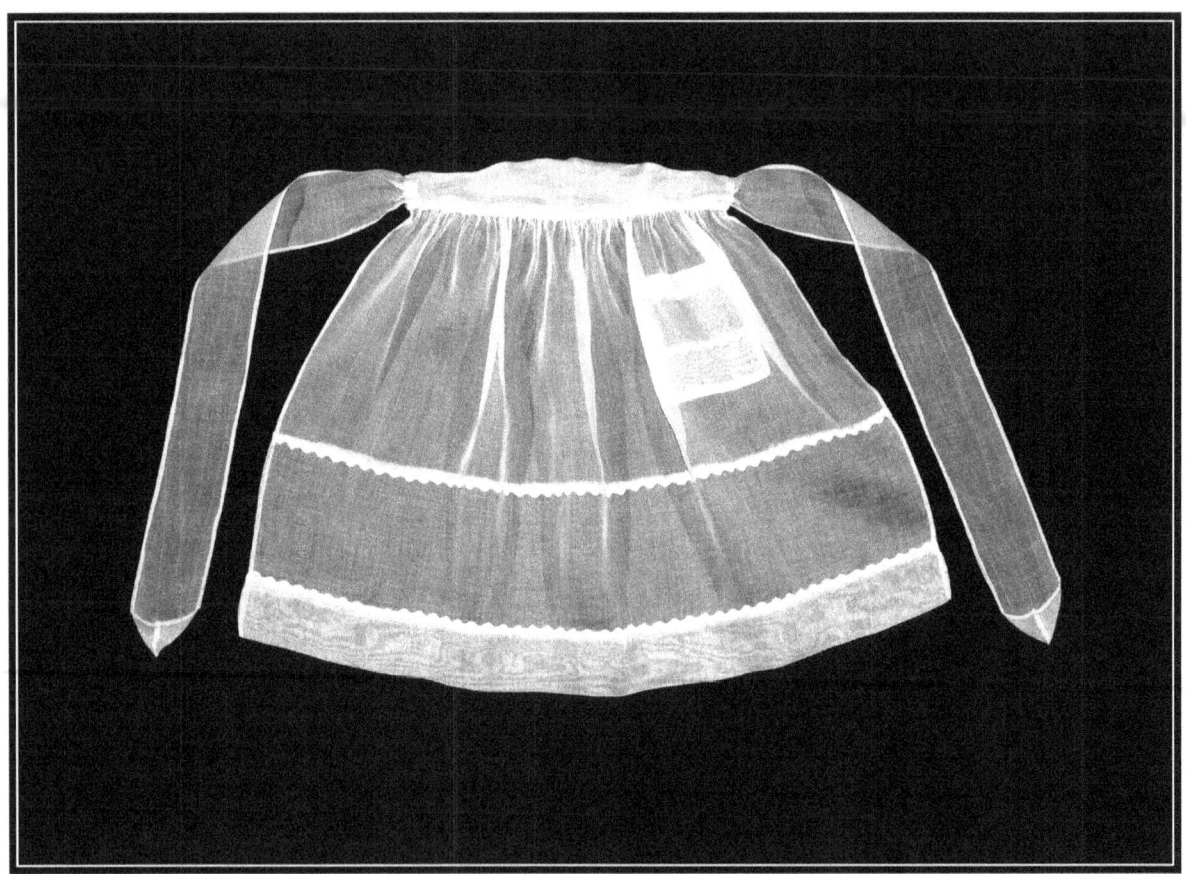

Adopted March 13, 2007 by Patricia Vuleta Spence Benn

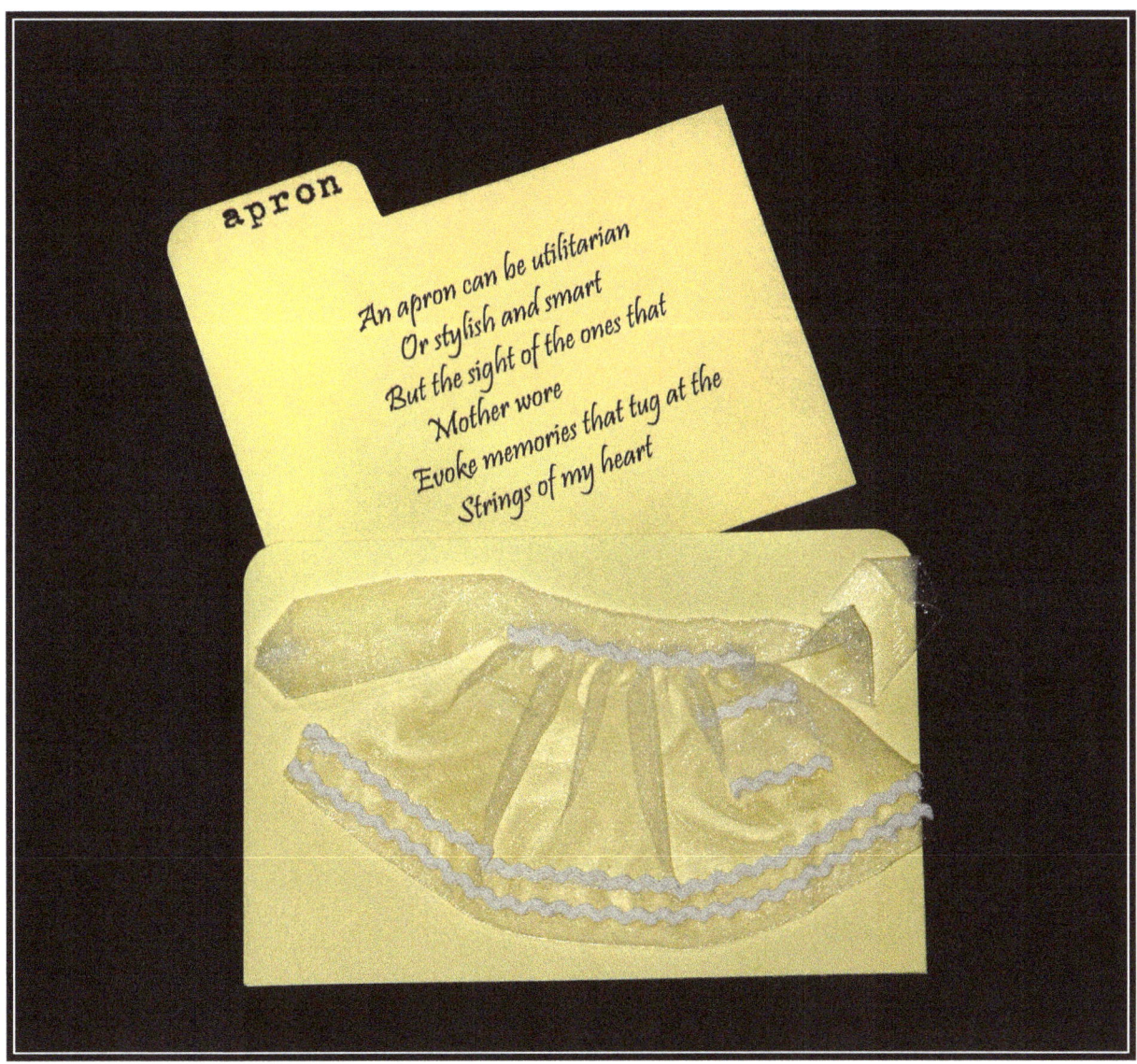

Pat Benn was inspired by her adopted apron to create this original recipe card

Gotcha Covered: A Legacy of Service and Protection

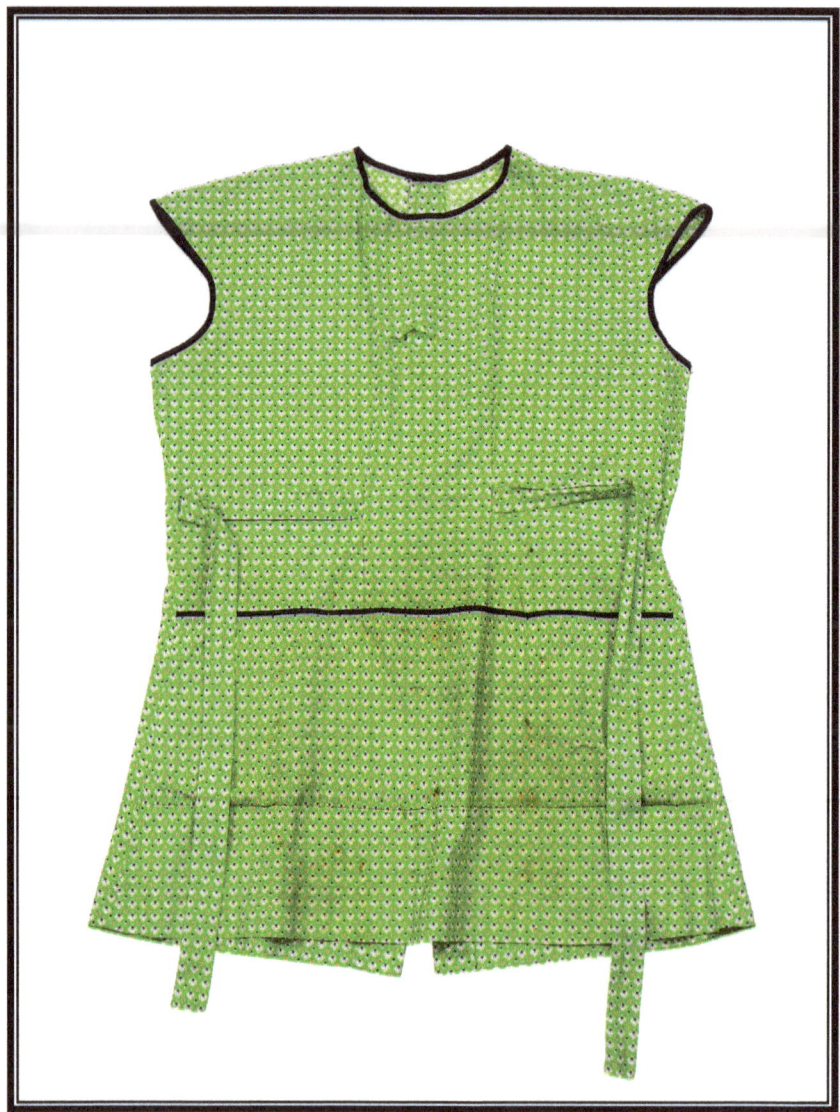

Adopted November 15, 2006 by Linda Scott Herzfeld

The Everyday Apron

Linda Scott Herzfeld

The everyday apron
        Worn and stained
                Memories of family fun
                        A mother's love.

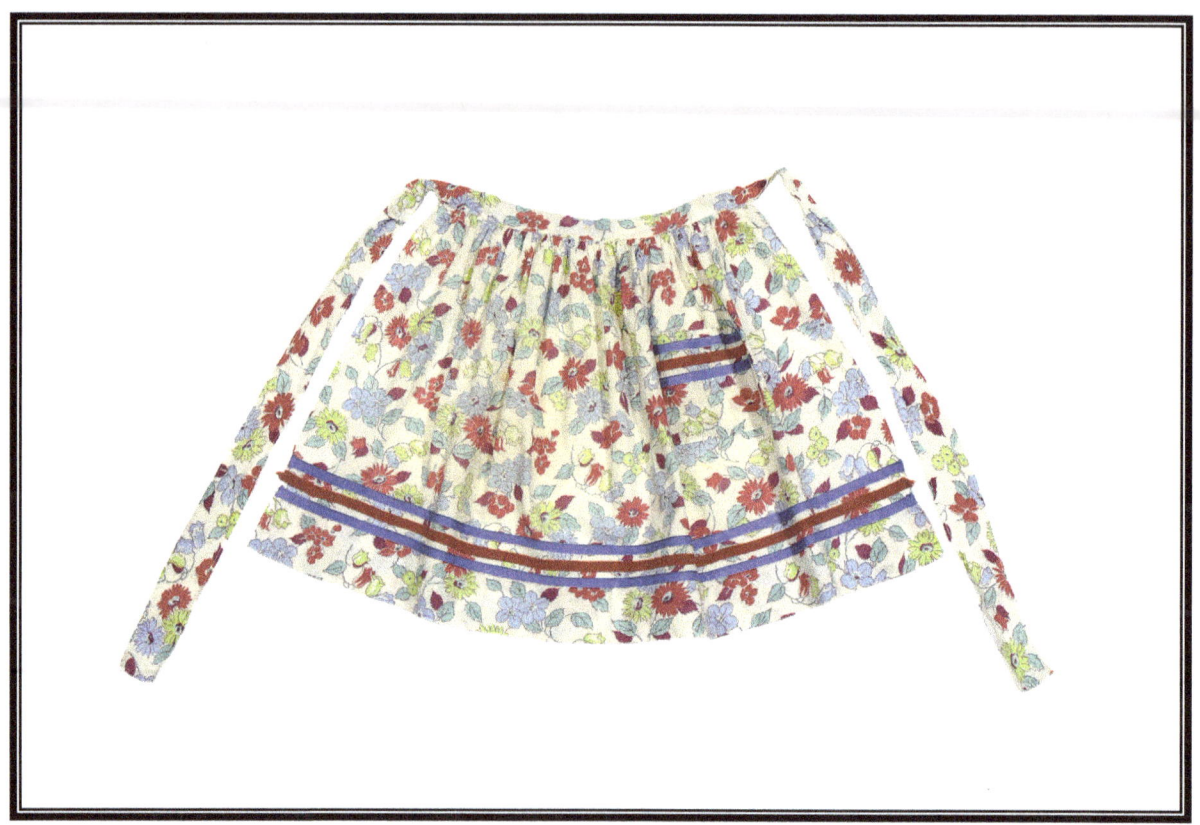

Adopted February 21, 2007 by Sharon Adkins

Mom

Sharon Adkins

Mom, you seem to be leaving a little more every day.
Conversations are vague; memory is fading.
Please stay a little longer.

Remember . . .
    Hankies left in your apron pockets . . . and in the chair cushions.
    Ten different kinds of Christmas cookies . . . Granny's recipes.
    The new Betty Crocker cookbook.
    Peas hidden under my plate and in my pockets.
    The Mother and Daughter Banquet.
    Rickrack trim on the aprons you made.
    Boiled potatoes . . . ALL the time.
    Flour-sack dishtowels and crocheted dishrags.
    The ladies of the church kitchen.
    Thanksgiving turkey leftovers stored in the attic.
    Spam-burgers.
    Church potluck dinners and lime Jell-O.
    Cream of mushroom soup . . . for everything.
    Oleomargarine in a bag.
    Hankies from your apron pocket . . . to wipe away my tears.
Mom, I love you.

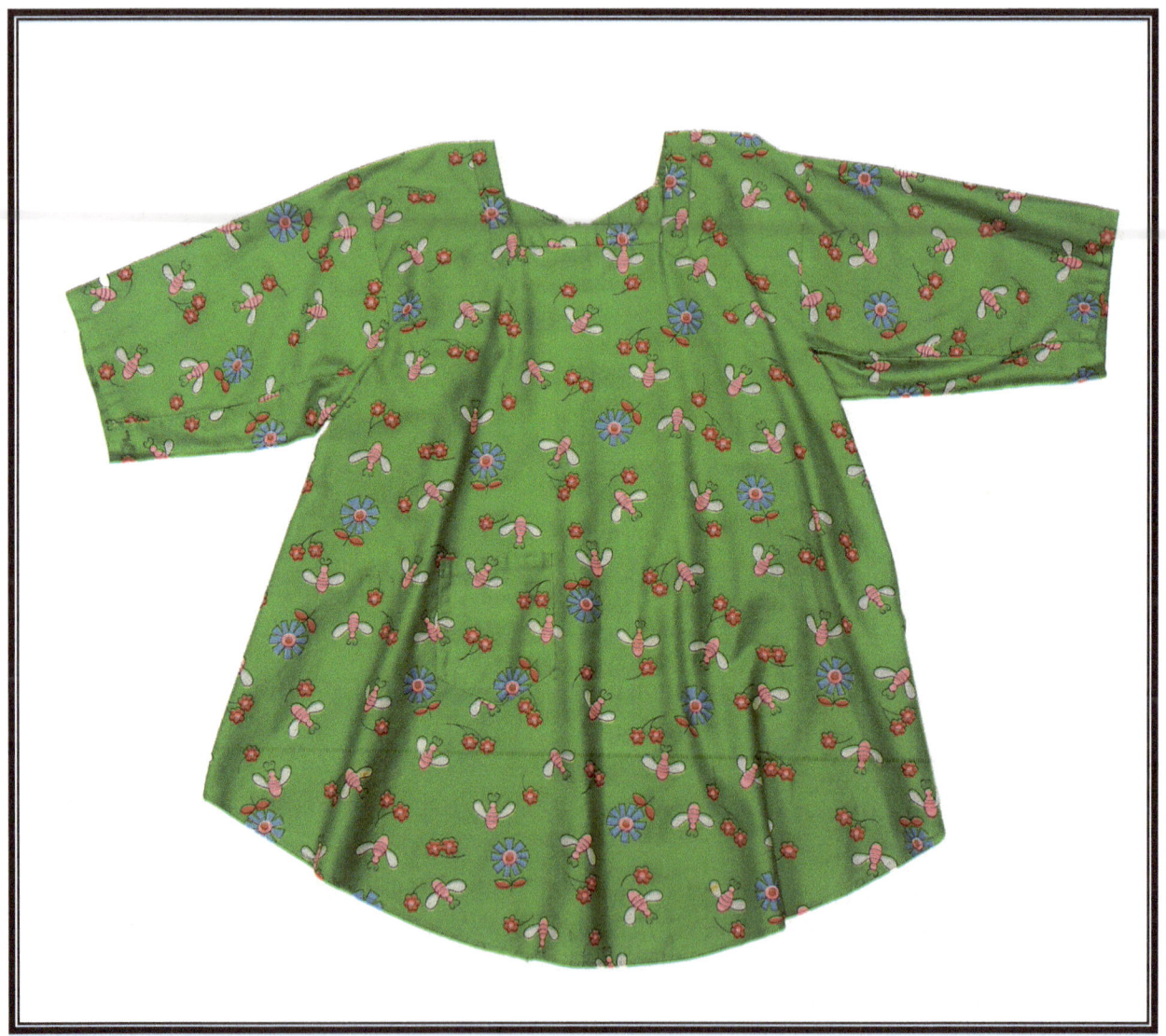

Adopted June 11, 2007 by Beverly Byram

Aprons

Beverly Byram

Aprons are a sweet link to my past. When I think of aprons I think of my great-grandmother. We called her Mamagran. Mamagran was a tall, stocky woman with long, gray hair, which she braided and pinned up on her head. She was strong, quiet, and kind. She loved to cook, tend African violets, and take care of her chickens. She loved children most of all.

An apron was a part of her daily wardrobe. She made her aprons out of colorful, floral prints that were soft to the cheek from many washings. The aprons had lots of pockets. The bounty of objects that appeared from those pockets met many varied needs. The things that she pulled out most, for me, were hankies and lemon gumdrops.

She died when I was sixteen. After forty years, I still have a windowsill full of African violets from her original plants. I wish I had one of her aprons, but at sixteen it never occurred to me that I would want one.

When I think of aprons I think of my Mamagran, and I smile.

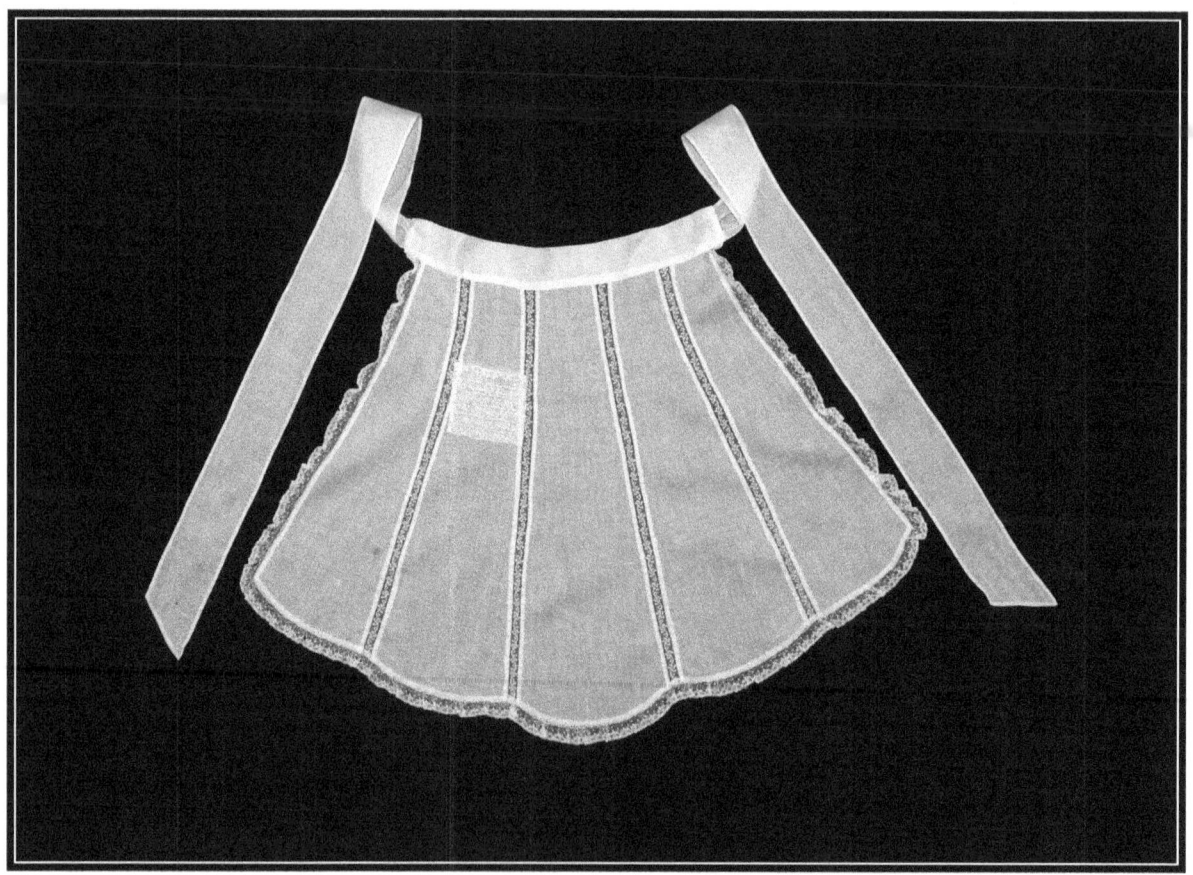

Adopted December 22, 2006 by Kathleen S. Lewis

Texanna Jones

Kathleen S. Lewis

When I look at this apron, I think of Texanna Jones . . . dark brown skin, a deep belly laugh, jolly brown eyes, rotund figure, huge smile on her face, wearing a black dress with a white apron over it. Anna—aka Texanna—my emotional and spiritual mother, came to work for my family when I was only a year old. My mother was bipolar and needed a maid to help her. Anna remained with us until my two older brothers and I had moved away from home. I was in my mid-twenties. By then, both my father and my only surviving grandparent, who lived with us, had died.

When I was leaving home after my father's death, I gave Anna a ride to her home. She reached over and put her hand on my arm and said, "Kathleen, don't yous worry now . . . I knows how to take care of your mama." Several years later, Anna was at the house with my mother. She clutched her chest with pain and fell into a chair in the den, where she had never been allowed to sit or lounge before. Anna died at the hospital a few days afterwards from a heart attack.

Memories of Anna flood my mind. She never did anything halfway. If a mouse appeared, Anna was on a stool screaming. A lightning and thunderstorm was endured in a walk-in, hall linen closet. She sang spirituals as she ironed, and said she was "raining" when perspiration drops fell from her forehead. When Anna got the news over the phone that one of her ten children had been murdered, she screamed "Oh, my Lordy" and collapsed into a chair, where she continued crying, moaning, and screaming over and over. Other of her children found similar deaths, much to Anna's sorrow.

I can remember as a small child telling her, "Anna, zip me up . . . zip me down . . . button me up . . . button me down." She was always there, patient, loving, helpful, and jovial, especially when I was sick. Anna could be tough when it was needed. My older brothers would get into knock-down, drag-out physical fights. Anna would break them up with a broom like a tornado, when needed. You just didn't make her mad. My mother knew not to upset Anna.

Life was rough for Anna. She walked and took the bus for many miles from her country home to our house. My parents finally got a car for her. She was as proud of that car as if it were a royal carriage. Anna's alcoholic, abusive husband would attack her on the lonely, dark country road to their home, to steal her paycheck. That was the only income for her and her many children. Anna carried a knife to fight him off. There were scars on her arms from some of those fights.

What Anna could do in the kitchen would melt in your mouth . . . corn bread, black-eyed peas, fried okra, fried chicken . . . I could go on and on. Anna couldn't read. Most of her recipes were from her memory, until Mother taught her to read. When my parents were building their dream house, they made sure Mother and Anna would have enough room to be able to navigate the kitchen together. I can still remember Anna taking a break, sitting on a stool in that kitchen, looking out through the front window at the Blue Ridge mountain range.

Our whole family attended Anna's funeral, traveling great distances to be there. We were there to be with her children—the children she left at home so she could come take care of us. They were seated in the front row. Since we were honored guests, we were asked to sit in the choir loft, in front of everyone. They all seemed to know each one of us from what Anna had told them. During the service, the children and members of her family would moan and yell out their grief for Anna. They would fall across the casket, cry and scream about their loss of Anna, and would offer prayers of thanks that she was their mama. It was hard to sit quietly with tears running down my face and hear their grief and loss pour out. I wanted to join them at the casket, with tears and cries of my loss. We sat stoically, taking in the whole picture. I grieved like they did, only quietly. I didn't realize for some time that I was also one of Anna's children, emotionally and spiritually. I belonged there at the casket, too.

Strangely enough, the day Anna died I was scheduled to speak at a community church function on race relations. Instead of my prepared comments, I gave a eulogy for Anna, through tears. I wish now I knew more of the details of Anna's life. A simple white apron will always remind me of her—my Anna.

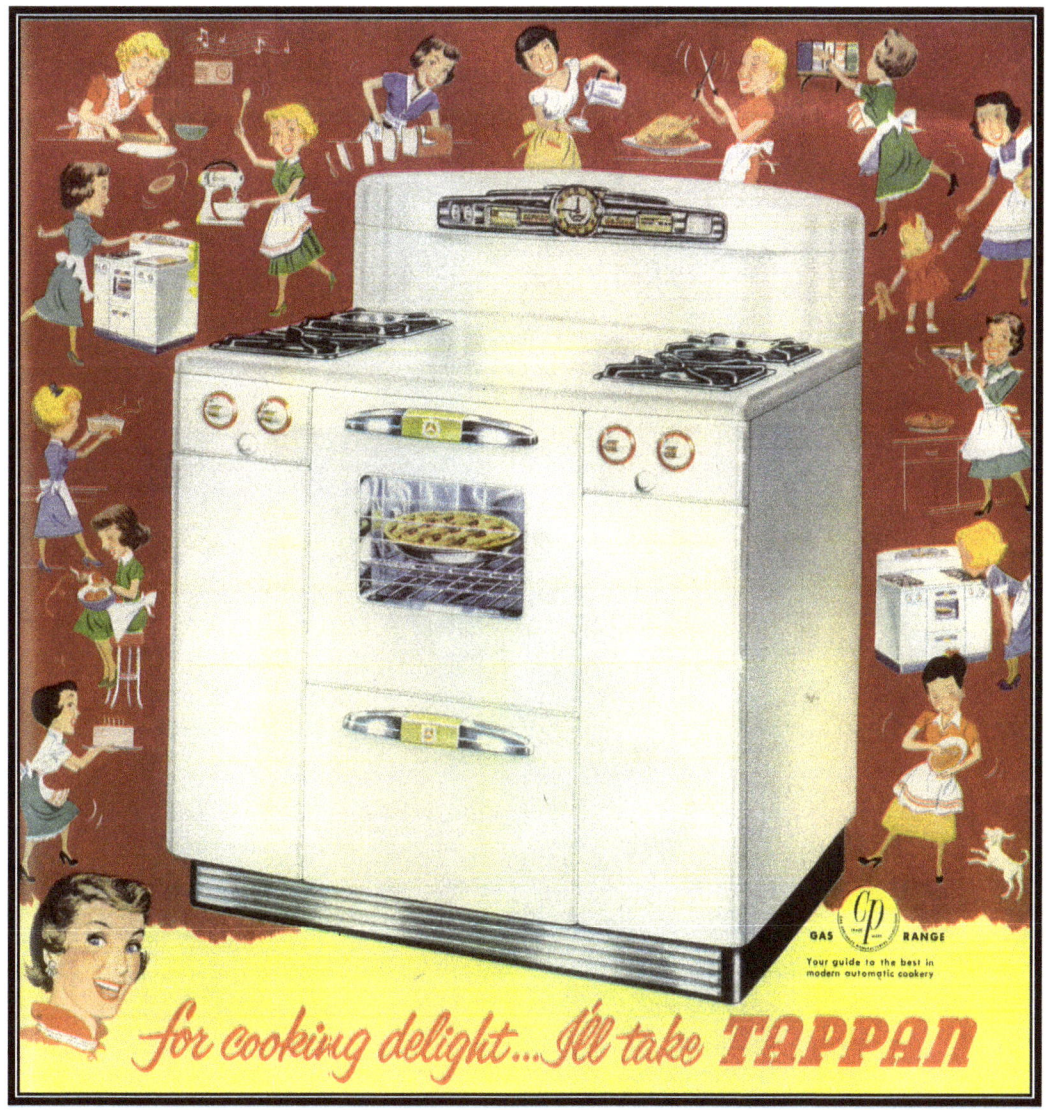

This advertisement for a Tappan range, which appeared in the March, 1952, *Better Homes and Gardens* magazine, shows all the roles for which women of the '50's might have been dressed in aprons—and of course, they are also wearing high heels and a smile. Image courtesy Electrolux.

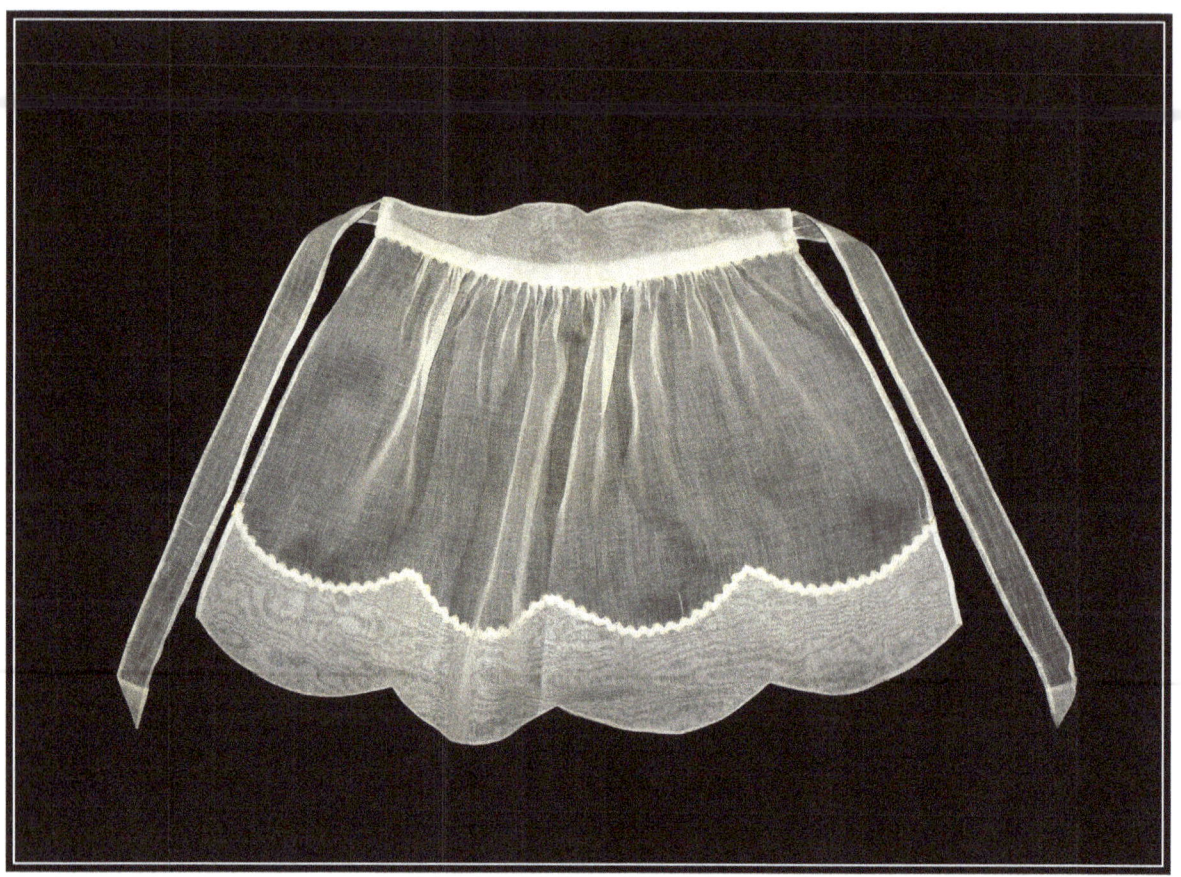

Adopted Spring 2007 by Dianne Horton Wood

A Cloud of Lavender-Blue

Dianne Horton Wood

Blue or lavender . . . always blue or lavender . . . predictable like the sunrise . . .

It was all about color: green garden, black walnuts, blue plates, yellow lemon pie, white bleached dish towels, red plums, blackberries. And there was the marvelous wooden kitchen utensil—with bright-red painted handles. She patiently wielded it back and forth, back and forth, back and forth.

"Honey, give Soo Soo another little bit of flour," she said, as she motioned for me to dip my tiny hands into the magical white stuff. Of course when I placed it on the table, it was with such flourish that a cloud of white dust rose. Never, ever did she say, "don't" or "no"—a safe and magical relationship that remained untarnished by the desire to discipline me.

She would always get up at 4:00 a.m., well into her seventh and eighth decade, just like she did when she got up to "make biscuits for Pa and the boys." So whenever I got to her house, she was well into her day. Wanting to spend her time with me, she had my breakfast ready and our lunch on by early a.m. But, if we were to have my special lunch of chicken and dumplings, she waited to wield the bright-red-handled rolling pin until I arrived. She was a cloud of lavender, interrupted only by her apron. She would roll the dumplings paper-thin, occasionally wiping her hands on a cloth or her apron. Into the boiling broth full of cut-up chicken and cooked eggs, she dropped the dumplings, along with a spoonful of butter the size of an egg. Soon, they were done. She set the table with a feast for us two, and took her apron off to signify time to eat.

In the afternoon, after the kitchen was cleaned, she changed to a good apron, a beautiful white cloud now joining the lavender one. She never wore a good apron until the afternoon, whenever she would go to sit in her rocker on the porch. There she told me stories of growing up in rural Mississippi at the turn of the century. She told of hard work on the farm. She told of her teaching career of forty years, teaching the first grade. She told of being one of the first women anywhere around to own a car, and many other wonderful tales she wove into my memory. The white apron floated in the slight breeze that blew across the porch. The only exceptions were the times that I sat in her lap while she rocked me, which she did until my feet touched the porch.

Later, we would go in and she would take my doll and cut out a new dress. "We will have to start on this next time, in the cool of the morning," she would say. She would stand on the porch in her beautiful lavender dress—always lavender—when my mother would come to gather me to go home. Her beautiful white apron would be blowing in the breeze until she was out of my sight.

I have a picture of her—my great-aunt Lucy—on her one-hundredth birthday. It sits beside my bed. It is the last thing I see at night before I meet her in my dreams.

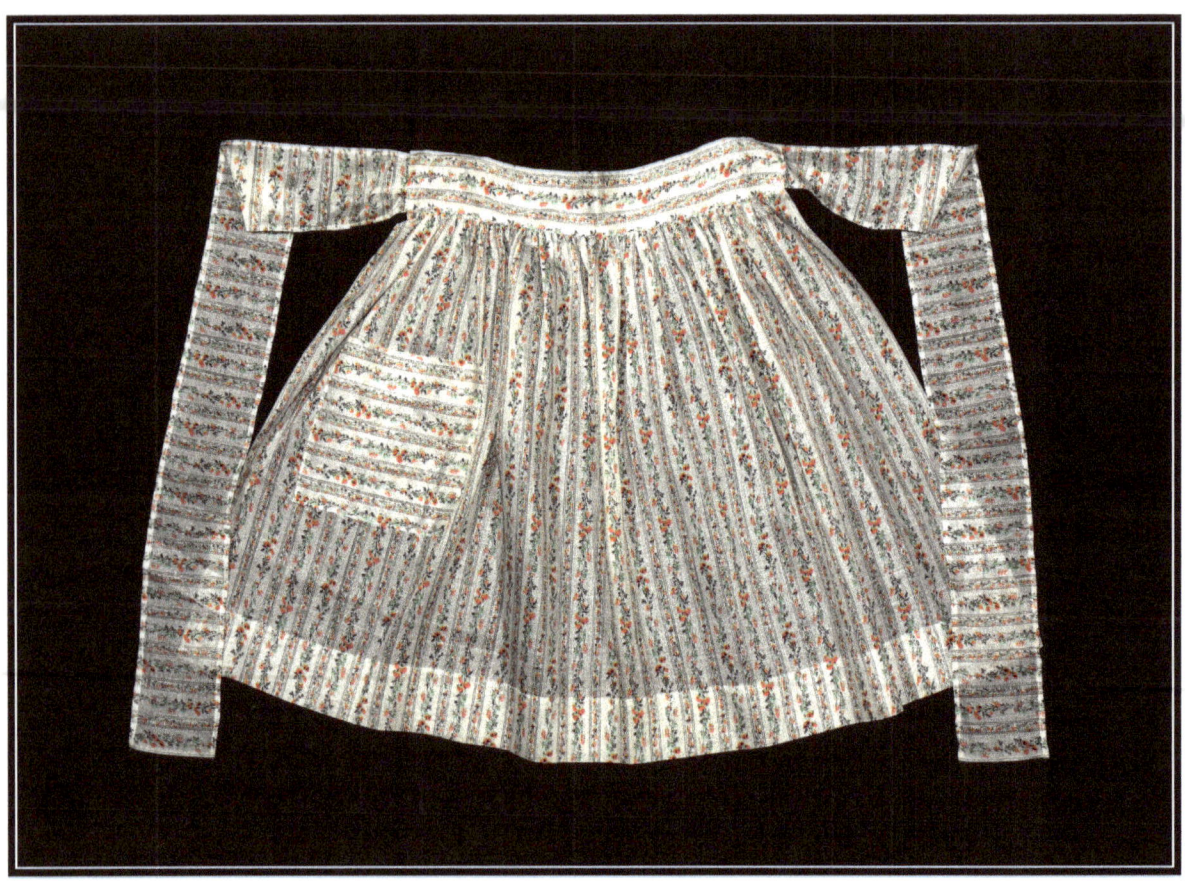

Adopted April 4, 2007 by Marceleen Rodes Alford

My Apron Memories

Marceleen Rodes Alford

During those tight-budget early years of marriage,
   my sewing machine made many a gift.
   Most treasured, by two Grandmothers, are their aprons,
 with the appliquéd handprints of each grandson.
Now in their nineties,
   the Grandmothers say,
"Plain, white, flour aprons for baking,
   frilly, trimmed aprons for Sunday dinner, and grandson-handprint aprons for love."

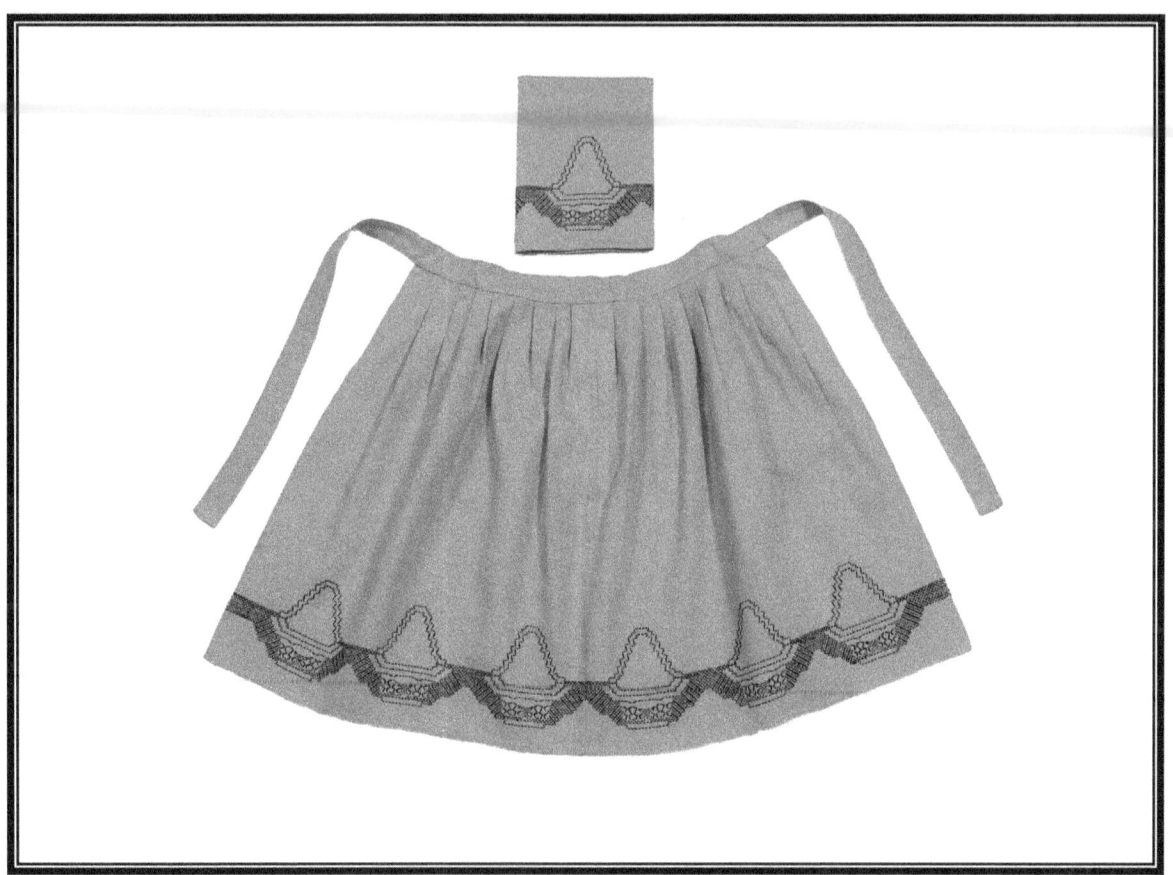

Adopted May 20, 2007 by Sue Wilson

Grandma's Aprons

Sue Wilson

Tying the long ribbons of fabric around my waist and smoothing the front of a delicately embroidered apron is like a step back in time. My apron, with its huck-weave embroidery, conjures images of Grandma's kitchen and the clatter, love, and taste of family.

I could smell the decadent aromas of the cinnamon rolls—Grandma's specialty—as the flavors melted together into gooey goodness in the oven. My sisters and I claimed we were waiting by the oven door to smell them as they baked. In reality, however, we jostled for position to be the first to sneak a pinch of the fresh treat as they emerged from the oven.

Grandma Agnes was a source of inspiration to us all. She was widowed at a young age, with five youngsters to raise and a farm to manage. As an adult, I look back and know that this couldn't have been an easy feat. As a child, I thought it was business as usual, as there was never a complaint from Grandma—only stories that made the things she baked seem even sweeter.

Grandma had many aprons, each for specific occasions. Her aprons were always pristine, having been washed in a wringer wash machine, then starched and ironed to perfection. Each apron had a unique design and a history lesson to go with it. We each had our favorite apron, and wearing them was like playing a lead role in the stories they represented. Grandma was a wonderful teacher. She not only taught us how to bake, to keep house, and to embroider our own apron, she also encouraged us to create our own story. I looked forward to the long days in her kitchen and the ride home with a car full of goodies and memories.

As each of us married and began our new life and our new stories, Grandma would arm each grandchild with the gift of a handcrafted apron, a rolling pin, and her special recipes, selected just for us. She said she hoped it would instill a passion for cooking and baking. I didn't spend the time in the kitchen that Grandma did, but I have passed her legacy on to my own girls and will continue to do so with my grandchildren. The rolling pin continues to be a staple in my kitchen, and I've committed most of the recipes to memory. But my grandmother's apron is tucked away, far too fragile to stand up to the kitchen today.

Grandma's apron strings wiped away many a tear as she listened, comforted, and encouraged us in her own remarkable way. Each grandchild was blessed by her hands, as she brushed the side of our young faces. Her legacy of faith, compassion, kindness, and love of family remain embedded in my heart. I thank God for Grandmas.

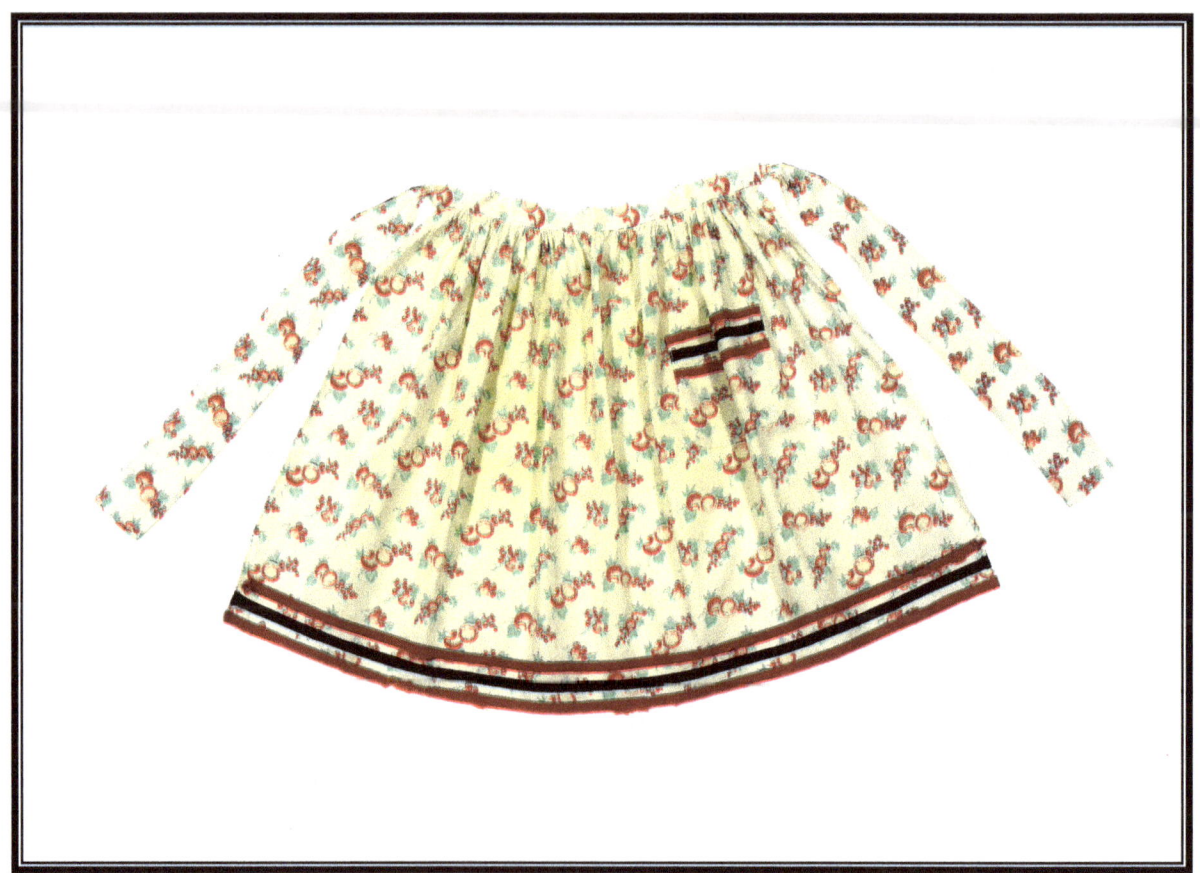

Adopted February 23, 2007 by Jennie Maddra Fleshood

Apron Images

Jennie Maddra Fleshood

Sometimes they were faded or spotty with food stains.

Other times, they were bright and bouncy or fresh and fancy—just for company.

Some covered the whole front of the wearer, neck to knee.

Others were small with a bow in back. These were just right for hand wiping.

Each apron seemed to express the personhood of the woman wearing it.

My mother's apron looked well-used and cheerful. It covered her whole front as she went about her daily chores.

Nanny's had fancy lacework and unusual designs. She loved to sew and cook, and her aprons seemed to say so.

Bubu's were small and bright and happy looking, just as she was. These aprons she wore only in the kitchen.

Mamie's aprons were frilly, in pastel colors. She wore them as she served Sunday dinners.

Aunt Jean's aprons were plain and simple. She wore them all day since she didn't like messes, and she seemed to clean a lot.

I made my apron as my first 4-H Club sewing project.

For the fabric, I used a pretty, multicolored "feedbag," which animal feed came in back then. I always felt grown-up and pleased with myself when I wore my "made by me" apron.

Because . . .

All the women I loved and knew best as a child wore aprons. Those aprons somehow defined the extraordinary place that each loved one has in my heart. Their aprons were a lovely part of them, and these women are so much a part of me.

Generational Legacies

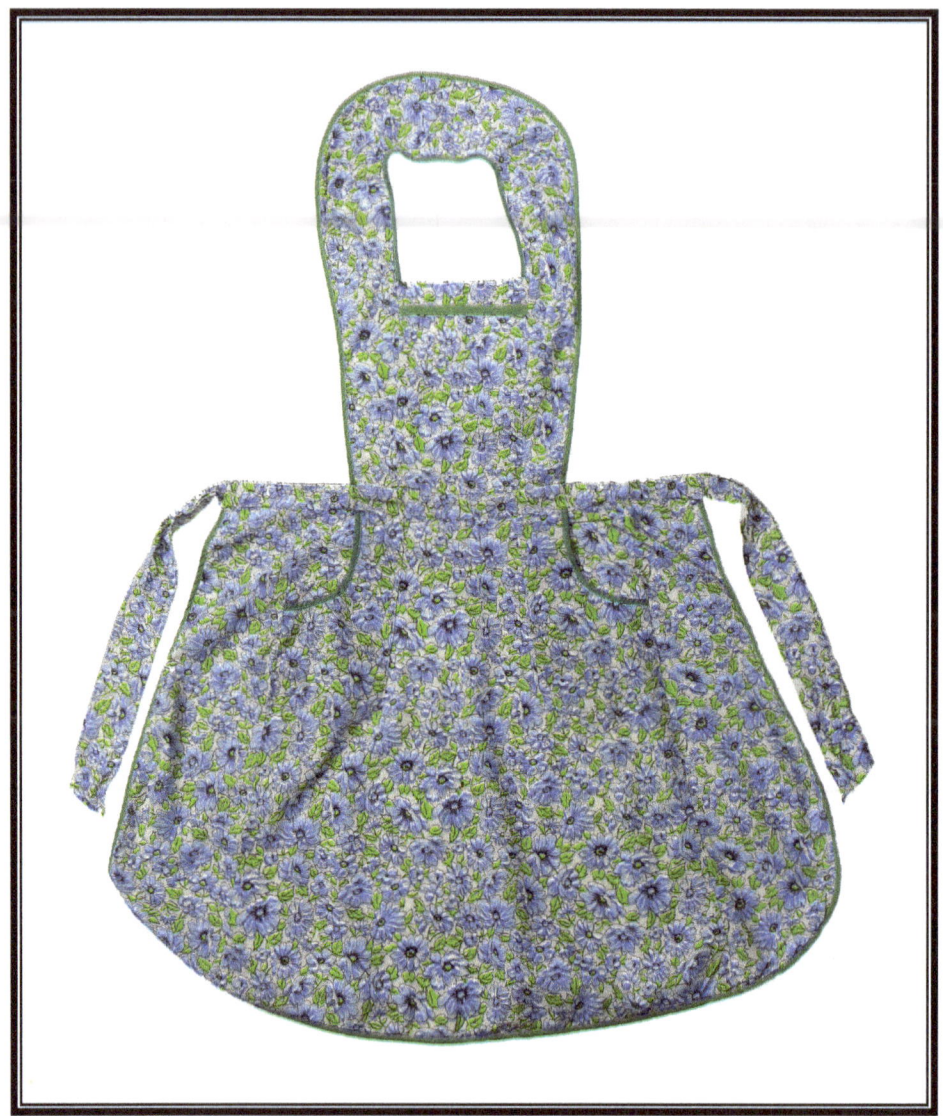

Adopted October 21, 2006 by Marilyn Hobbs McAtee

The Apron Interview

Marilyn Hobbs McAtee

The apron which I chose reminded me of both my Indiana mother and my Mississippi grandmother—bib-style, blue flowers, deep pockets, handmade, simple, functional but beautiful. Both my mother and my grandmother wiped their hands on aprons, but both also wiped away the tears of a daughter and granddaughter.

On New Year's Eve 2006, as I was making edible lips in my kitchen with Taylor, my six-year-old granddaughter, and her friends, Morgan, six, and Hannah, nine, I interviewed them about aprons. Taylor calls me "Big Mama"—I am a fourth-generation Big Mama—a Southern thing.

Big Mama: "What do aprons look like?"
Taylor: "They are kind of like dresses, except they have spaghetti strings and they tie."
Morgan: "Some can be in different colors."
Hannah: "You can wear an apron for dress-up."
Taylor: "They come in good and handy."
Morgan: "Aprons make our clothes not get dirty."
Hannah: "An apron comes in handy so you can cook."
Taylor: "Aprons make you nice and clean."
Hannah: "They are also handy so you don't get paint on your clothes."
Big Mama: "Who wears aprons?"
The girls: "Chefs, cookers, grandmas, grandpas, moms, and dads."
Hannah: "Are we going to be published? I wrote the recipe for the lips."
"START COOKING! THE END."

God Bless Our Little Ones.

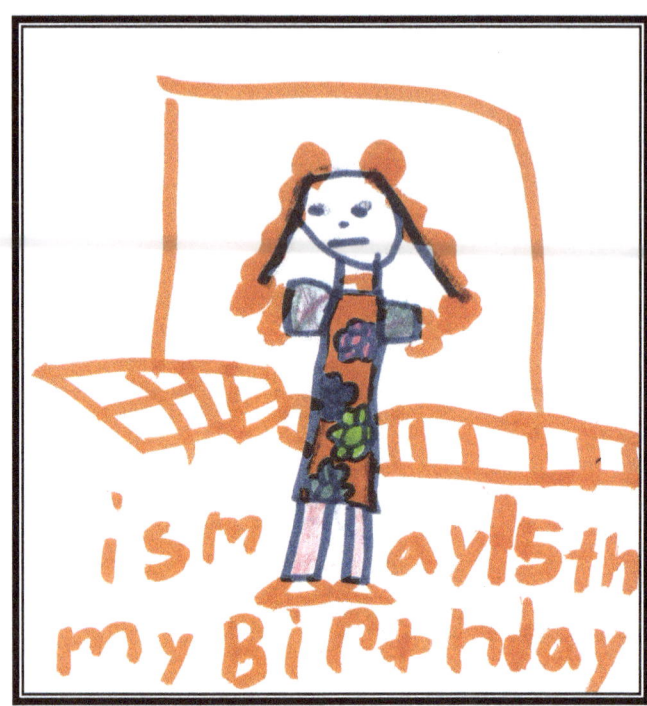

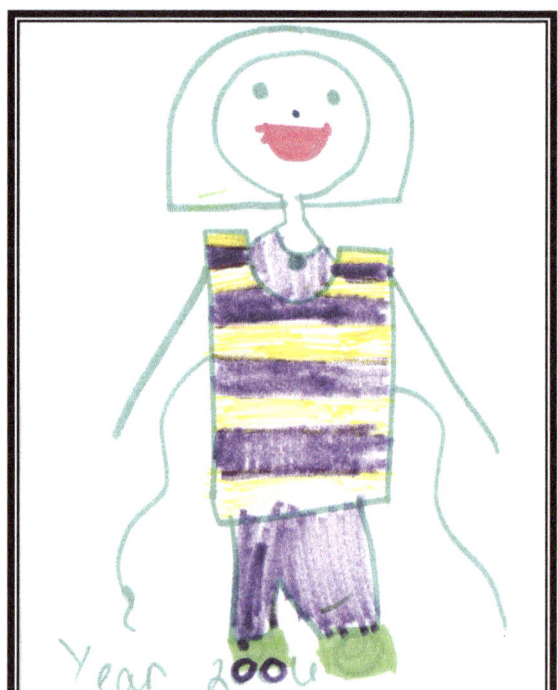

Taylor Politan's self-portrait in an apron, noting her birth date.
(Submitted by Taylor Politan)

Hannah Cozzolino self-portrait, wearing an apron.
(Submitted by Hannah Cozzolino)

Hannah Cozzolino added a "bonous" page recipe for Edible Lips to her apron-clad self-portrait. (Submitted by Hannah Cozzolino)

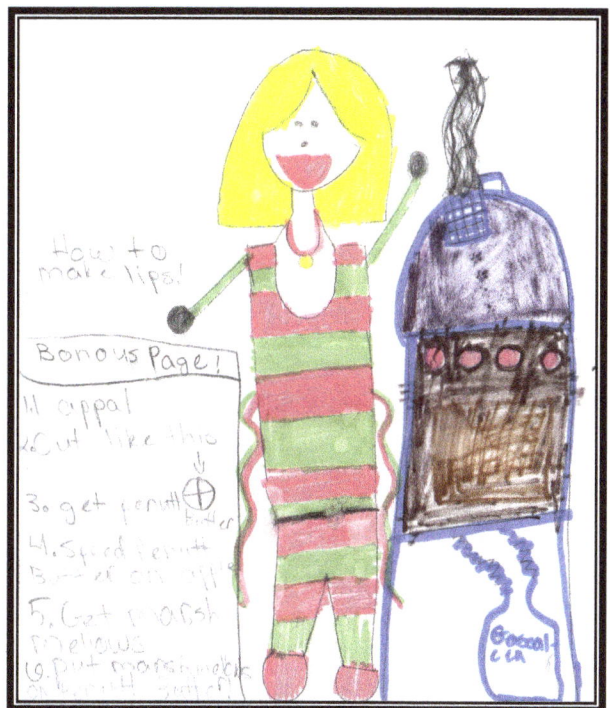

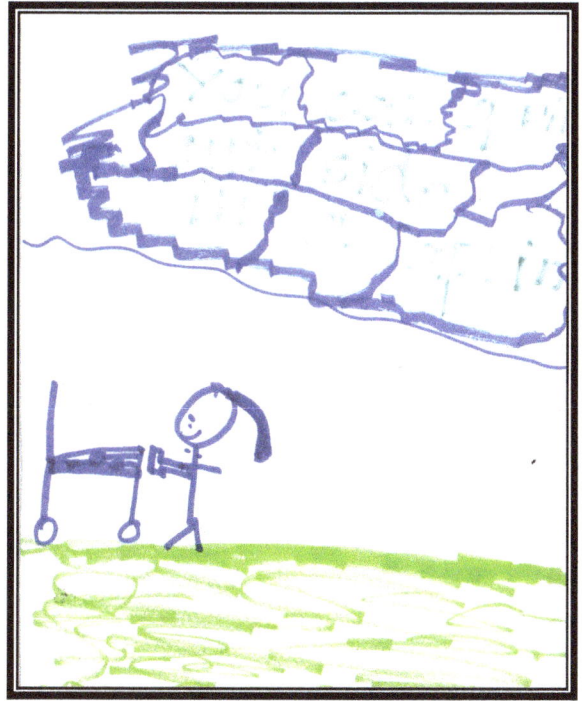

Morgan Cozzolino explains, "You can grill outside in a aprin." (Submitted by Morgan Cozzolino)

GOTCHA COVERED: A LEGACY OF SERVICE AND PROTECTION

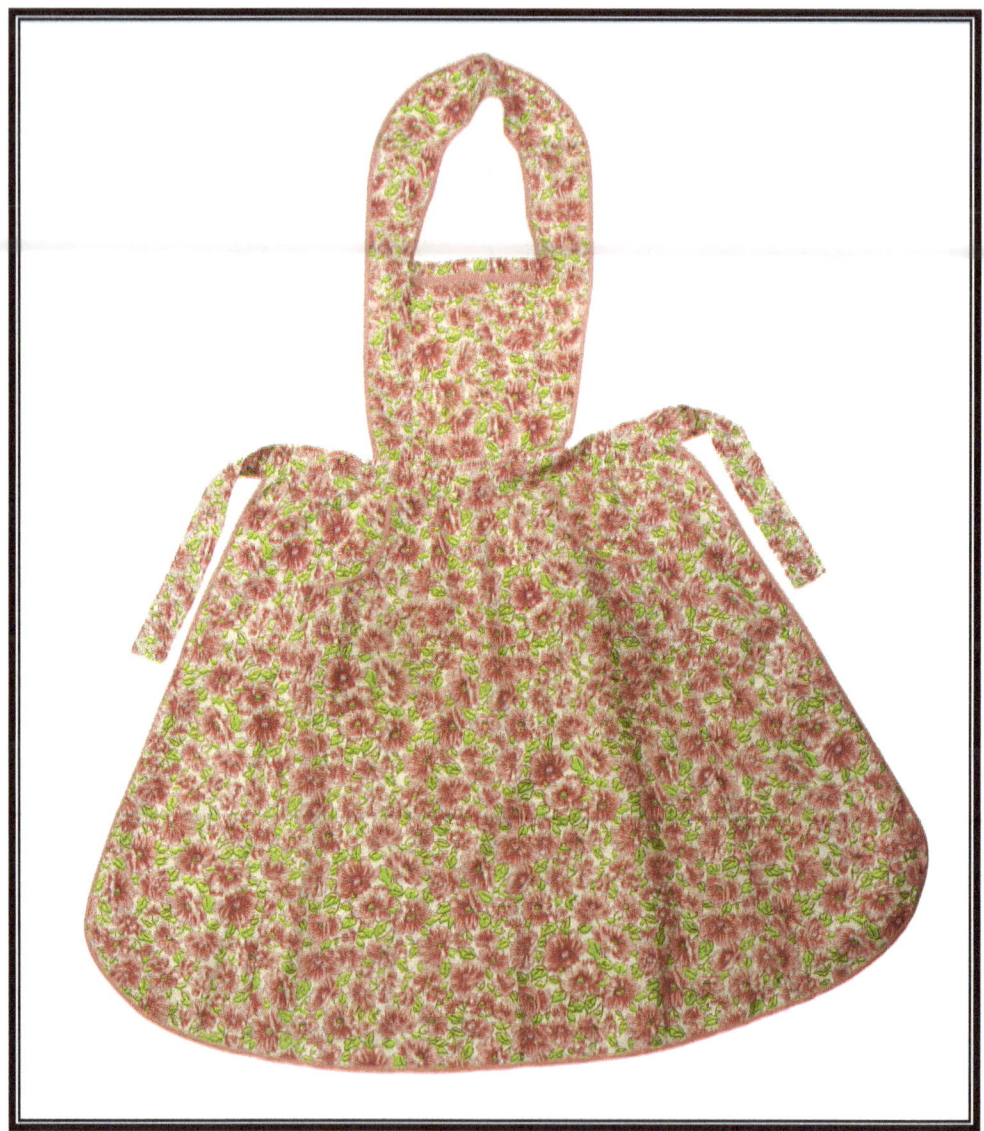

Adopted December 20, 2006 by Libby Dayani

Apron Memories

Libby Dayani

I'm old enough to have fond memories of aprons—those of my mother and of both my grandmothers. There was a time when cooking and sharing mealtimes were treasured, shared, family activities. These times provided vital physical and spiritual nourishment, and cherished memories.

My mother learned to cook from scratch from her mother. In turn, Mother taught me how to cook from scratch. And of course, we always wore an apron—either a frilly one for teas or bibbed ones for serious cooking. When I baked my first cake from scratch, I forgot to add the vanilla. Recognizing my mistake, I pulled the cake out of the oven, stirred in the vanilla, and shoved the pan back in the oven. Needless to say, the cake turned out flat as a pancake. My creative mother proceeded to make a pudding, and then she cut up the cake and poured the pudding over it. Voila! We had a delicious pudding cake. I experimented a lot, and she never scolded me for any cooking failures.

On Saturdays and Sundays, at my maternal grandmother's home, she would don an apron long before we were out of bed. She prepared a breakfast feast—scrambled eggs, salt mackerel, sausage and bacon, fried apples in season, and homemade biscuits. Her Sunday and holiday dinners were just as wonderful. I still have her recipe for Christmas Lane Cake and ambrosia made from scratch. We sat for hours peeling and sectioning fresh oranges. Does anyone take that time anymore? Half the joy was sitting in the kitchen shelling peas, stringing beans, or peeling oranges, and talking while the intoxicating aroma of delicious foods swirled through the house.

Sometimes on Sunday evening, instead of a meal, Mother would have a "tea." This included toast fingers with cream cheese and jam, and tea with cream and sugar. To this day, I love to have tea. Every Sunday, we would use her fine china, crystal, and sterling flatware. We learned good manners and good conversations at an early age.

My paternal grandmother also used aprons. Everyone did in those days, but she wasn't a great cook. However, she bought wonderful, store-bought goods, so it seemed like a special treat to eat the Hostess donuts, cookies, and cakes that we didn't get at home. When your food and clothes are homemade, you think that store-bought items are better, until you are old enough to know better.

My Dad wasn't much of a cook either, but I do remember him making Concord grape and pineapple jam a couple of times. He also loved to garden, and he and Mom would can the extra tomatoes and make cucumber pickles.

At this time in my life, I am returning to cooking from scratch, although I modify the recipes to be healthier. We know more about nutrition now. No more lard or fatback. I love knowing that when I wear the aprons I inherited from the women in my life, I am savoring and passing on the love they so generously gave to me when they wore theirs.

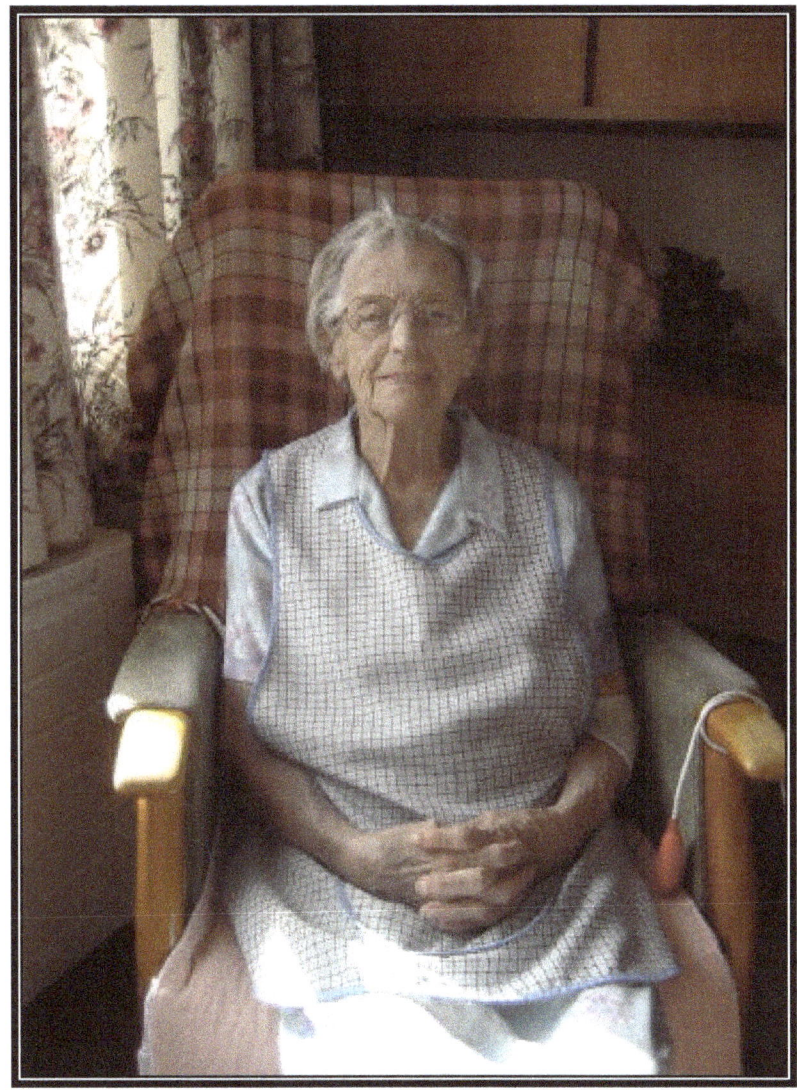

Mrs. May Graham lives in the Retired Nurses' National Home in Bournemouth, Dorset, U.K. She was a nursing officer in a psychiatric hospital and in her retirement she wears an apron every day. Photo submitted by Eileen Richardson.

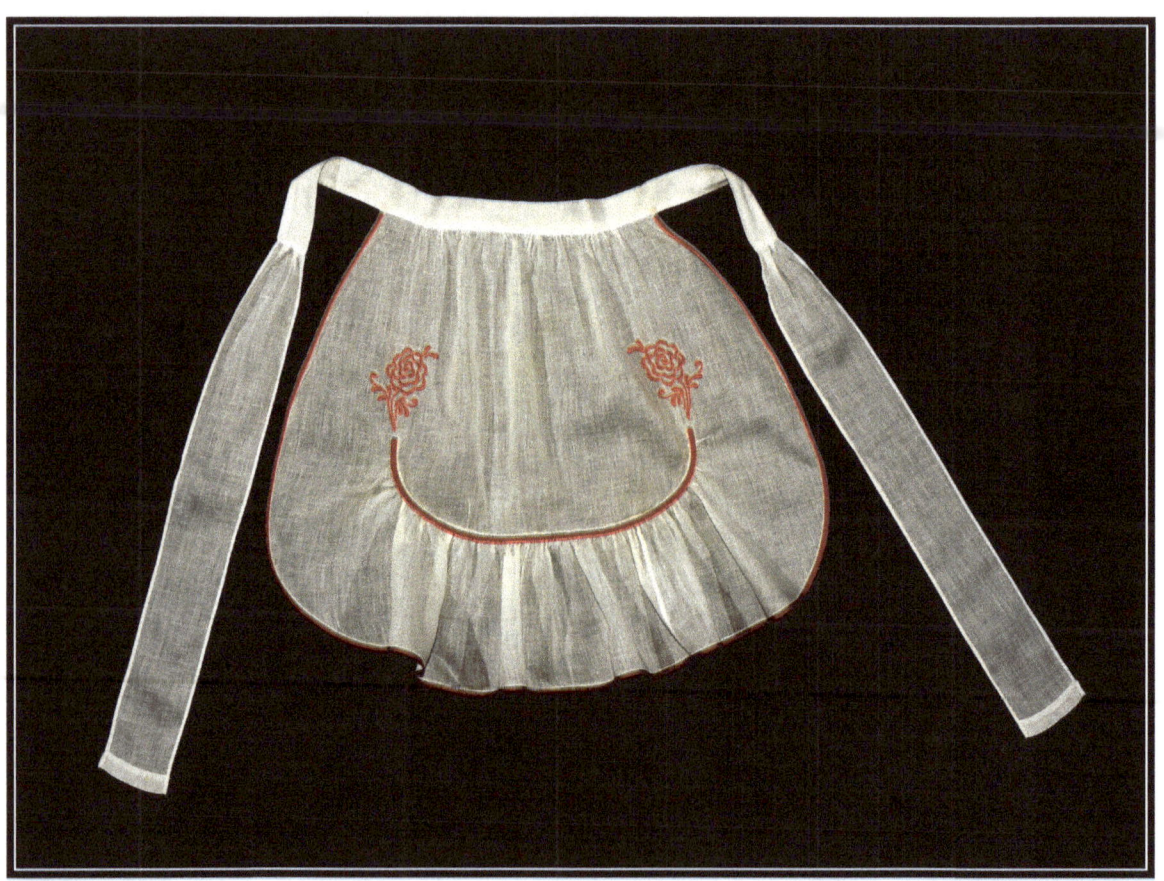

Adopted November 4, 2006 by Charlotte Richardson Norwood

Aprons... Ties... Traditions... Changes... Generations

Charlotte Norwood's granddaughters live in China with their parents. While visiting in Virginia, they were photographed by their grandfather wearing Charlotte's adopted apron.

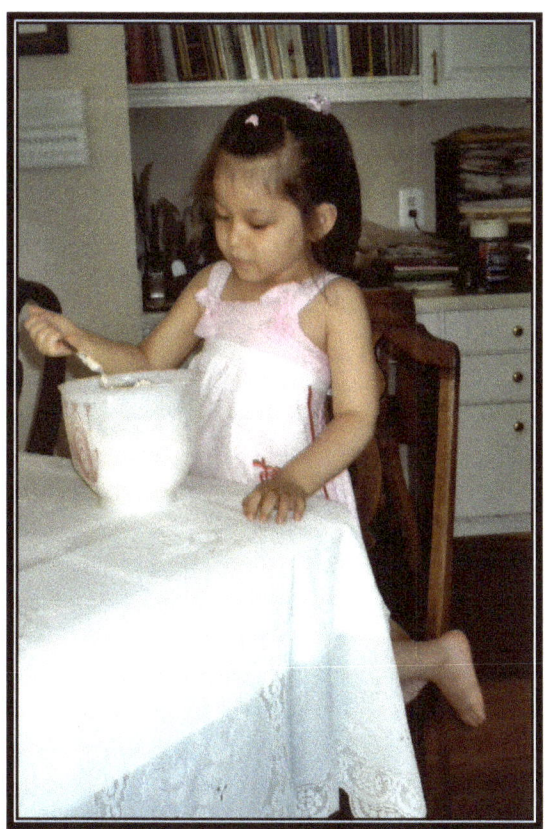

Freya Norwood

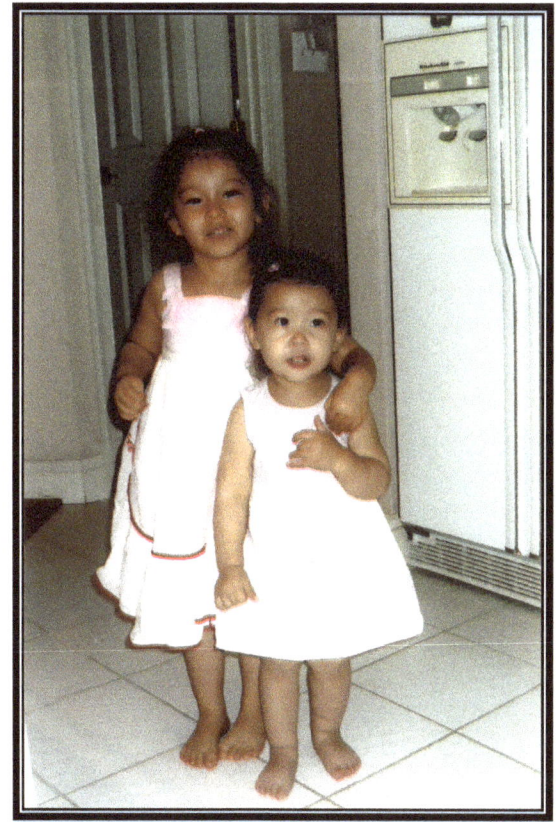

Freya and Alana Norwood.

(Photos courtesy of Thomas Norwood)

PART FOUR: *Aprons as Symbols of Imagination and Creativity*

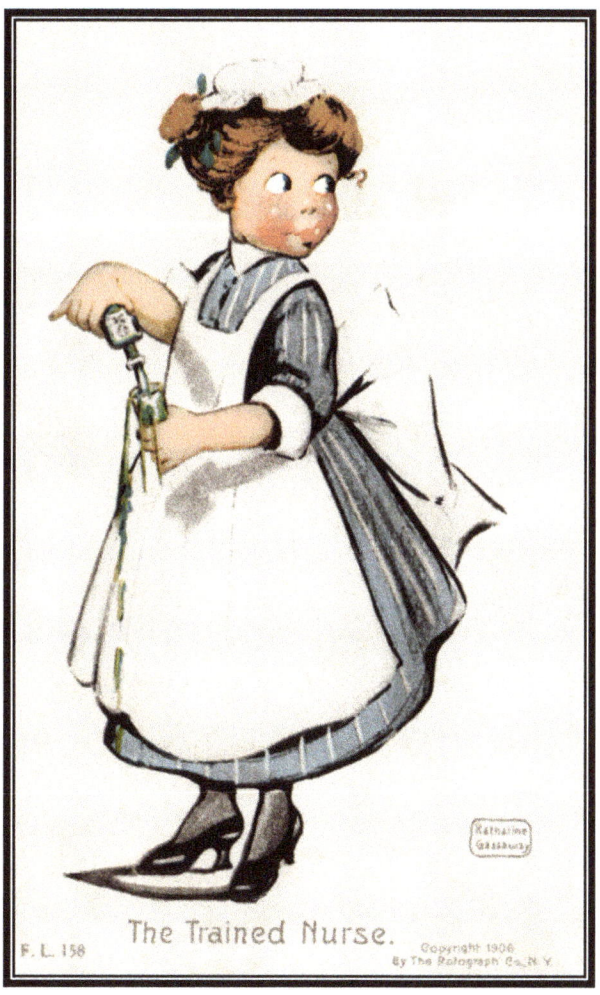

© Zwerdling Nursing Archives, used with permission.

Aprons as Symbols of Imagination and Creativity

Ginger T. Manley

The minute I tie on my apron, I feel ready for adventure. It is like the exact moment in Field of Dreams *when the young ballplayer crosses over the line and becomes an aging country doctor again.*

Marcy Goldman www.betterbaking.com

Aprons have been favorite tools as prompts for writers for thousands of years. A quick Internet search turns up these examples:

The coarse satiric poem *Pleasant Quippes for Upstart New-fangled Gentlewomen (1595)*, attributed to the English writer Stephen Gosson says:

These aprones white of finest thred
So choicelie tide, so dearlie bought,
So finely fringed, so nicelie spred,
So quaintlie cut, so richlie wrought,
Were they in worke to save their cotes,
They need not cost so many grotes. ("Aprons in the Middle Ages and Renaissance")

William Shakespeare's frequent use of aprons in his plays has fueled discussion about the possibility of his having been a Freemason. Two examples cited in support of this conclusion include: "Here, Robin, as I die I give thee my apron." (*Henry VI*. II, 2:14), and "A carpenter—where is thy leather apron and thy rule?" (*Julius Caesar* I, 1:7) (Clegg)

Medieval artists have left abundant painted images of people wearing aprons, including a particular style of apron worn by midwives in fifteenth-century Germany and Austria, in which "the aprons' [*sic*] strings come up to the woman's shoulders, and it seems to cover both the front and the back." ("Aprons in the Middle Ages and Renaissance") In her book, *Nursing: The Finest Art* (1985), M. Patricia Donahue published hundreds of artistic renderings of nurses and healers from primitive to modern times. Two images of nurses wearing aprons, "The Attentive Nurse" (p. 29) and "A Medieval Hospital" (p. 120), show the role aprons have played throughout history in artistic depictions of healing.

While not a fictional event, Lizzie Borden is quoted from court records about the murder of her parents, "I had no occasion for an apron that morning." ("Lizzie Andrews Borden quotes")

In a seventeenth-century version of English property-rights law, a man was given authority to use, for himself, his wife's inherited real estate during her lifetime, thereby tying himself metaphorically to her apron strings. Over time, writers have attached feelings of disdain and feelings of longing to the expression "apron strings." Anne Brontë, writing in *The Tenant of Wildfell Hall* (1848), uses the phrase pejoratively in chapter three when Mrs. Markham scolds her guest, Mrs. Graham, for spoiling her young son by bringing the child along for a visit. "Even at *his* age, he ought not to be always tied to his mother's apron string; he should learn to be ashamed of it." (Brontë, p. 26)

Elvis Presley has been characterized as being tied to the apron strings of his mother. In his case, the phrase indicates his excessive devotion to his mother, rather than his dependence on her property. Apron-string connections were significant enough to him that he recorded the hit song "Apron Strings," ("'Apron Strings' lyrics") in which he repeats in each refrain his wish to be tied to the apron strings of his hoped-for lover. Later, when he was seeking a birthday gift for Lisa Marie, he commissioned the poem, *The Priceless Gift* (McComb, 1971), which is now framed and hanging in the kitchen at Graceland. The poem tells the story of Elvis finding an apron belonging to his mother in an old trunk in the attic and giving the apron to Lisa as a symbol of her grandmother's love.

In the historical novel, *Girl with a Pearl Earring* (Chevalier, 1999), set in Delft in the 1600s, Griet, the protagonist, wears an apron as part of her housemaid's dress and as helper to the painter, Vermeer. The apron plays a key role in moving the plot forward in several scenes, like when a malevolent child sullies the apron as a way of attempting to place Griet in a bad light.

Aprons are worn in the United States as part of costumes for staging historical reenactments and for Halloween attire, sometimes as a naughty nurse. Female Civil War reenactors are encouraged to put a little dried blood on their aprons, to heighten the impression of having been on the battlefield. Patterns for constructing costume aprons are widely available for both girls and women who may be portraying Florence Nightingale, Dorothea Dix, or other historical nurse figures. In England, aprons are often worn by cross-dressing males, as part of fancy-dress costumes for New Year's Eve parties.

Dr. Jennifer Craik, a historian in Australia, informs us that "the cultural life and politics of this mundane garment are explosive." (Craik, 2006) Dr. Craik illustrates her point with an example from the research of Avis Smith, who toured Australia with her collection of vintage aprons, often giving talks before groups of women. When the audience would realize that one of Smith's aprons, purchased from an adult entertainment shop, was an adaptation of the very proper and almost invisible domestic apron worn by housemaids, but now embellished to suggest possible titillating sexual experiences, the attendees would become both amused and embarrassed. The transformation of the sedate parlor apron into one "so redolent of a sex life" (Craik, 2006) that it strikes an instant chord in its viewers reminds us again of the power of this humble garment to transport us from reality to fantasy.

Similarly, since the early 1980s, the historical white or striped apron of the nurse or candy striper has been converted by advertisers, filmmakers, and the porn industry into a vehicle of fantasy. Indeed, nurses have been targeted and exploited as objects of sexual fantasy more frequently than have any other occupational group.

The English author, Betty Neels (1911–2001), a registered nurse and midwife, had a thriving career after her retirement from nursing, writing more than one hundred Harlequin Romance novels, in which the female protagonist was often a nurse who has an encounter with a physician. One of her first books, published in 1970, was originally titled *Amazon in an Apron*, and then later retitled *Nurse in Holland*. (Neels) By current standards, the stories are actually quite tame compared to the lusty-sounding titles.

Geraldine Pearson recently reviewed the novel *Aprons on a Clothesline* (DePree, 2005) for the nursing journal, "Perspectives in Psychiatric Care" (Pearson, 2005). The story takes place in a small town in rural Minnesota where, as Pearson describes the protagonist, Virginia Morgan is "well-known to the townspeople as figuratively wearing an apron at all the occasions that involve 'doing'." Pearson suggests the story of Virginia and her family, coping as they do with Virginia's debilitating stroke, teaches important lessons for nurses.

Aprons—powerful vehicles for inspiring fantasy, creativity, fiction, and nonfiction.

Fiction

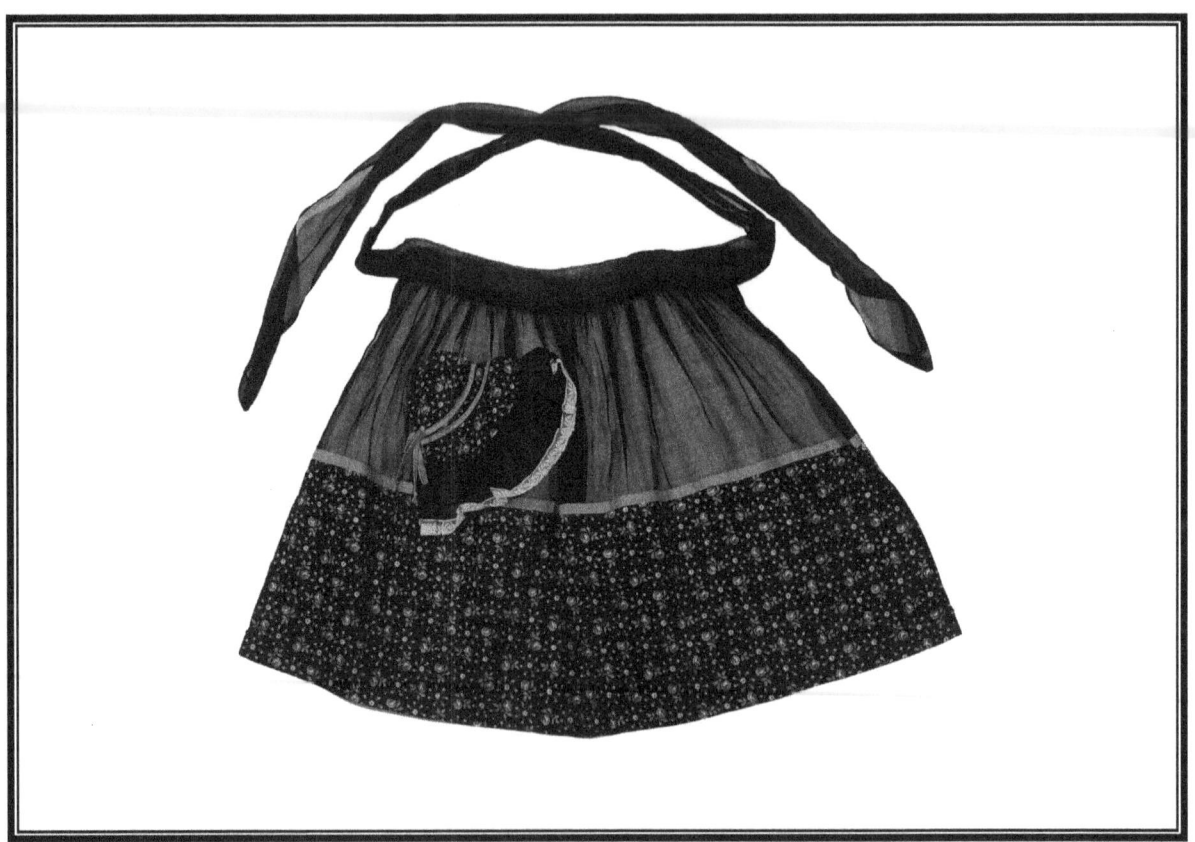

Adopted October 28, 2006 by Suzanne Hopkins Blievernicht

Nothin' Says Lovin'

Suzanne Hopkins Blievernicht

"Honey, pull out my underwear drawer and see if you can wear any of my panties. I bought a bunch of new ones just before I had to start wearing Depends. I hate it that they are just lying there in the drawer."

It was late morning and they sat in her bedroom sipping coffee. The winter sun, in its lower orb, cast a warm glow on her mother as she stretched out for her ritual sunbath on the peach-silk boudoir chair in front of the large picture window. Her feet were perched on a black velvet ottoman and covered with a bright pink afghan.

"Mama, are you sure? I don't want to start pawing through your stuff."

"Listen, sweetie, it will be the Second Coming before either June Allison or I will ever wear them. Besides, they are nice Vanity Fair panties and they'll just rot otherwise. If you don't want them, take them to Goodwill. Besides, wouldn't you have fun emptying my drawers of my drawers?"

Both giggled.

All the daughter could think about was how her father's underwear still lay in the drawers on his side of the massive Italian Provincial dresser. His closet was a mess, the way he'd left it. It was his domain; the dresser was her mother's. It was she who folded his shirts and boxers, all facing the same direction like soldiers frozen in formation. The socks, in navy, brown, and black platoons, had not budged since they had come to an abrupt parade rest a decade earlier. These intimate parts of her father's wardrobe were some of the last vestiges of control remaining in her mother's rapidly narrowing world. Her mother had been insistent. If none of her sons wanted their father's things, they were not to be touched. "I'll do it later," she had promised. The daughter had resigned herself to reality. The gathering and disposal of both parents' underwear would be her responsibility, just as probably almost everything else would fall upon her and her sister later on. She didn't want to force the issue now. Her mother was taking a big step even offering her panties. Besides, this would lessen her own grief when the time came.

Carpe diem!

The daughter opened the middle dresser drawer on her mother's side and viewed the precisely stacked bras, panties, slips, and girdles. There were only two colors in her mother's lingerie repertoire—mostly white and a few black. Once, she had tried to talk her into flesh tones, but her mother had insisted on the old standby whites. Nudged to try underwire bras, she consented and agreed they gave her a perkier look.

"Okay, Mama. I'll have a look at what's in here and see what fits."

"Just the panties, honey. I may not have much bladder control, but I sure as hell am not going to let these girls hang out without a bra. They have a mind of their own!"

They laughed as the daughter shifted the bras carefully to one side of the drawer and pulled the plain white polyester panties forward. She held up her mother's lone black long-line bra, and a thigh-length black girdle, both always worn under her favorite evening dresses.

"Those sure have had a lot of fun times," said her mother.

Blindly, the daughter reached back into the drawer and swept the deep corners.

"Mama, there's something else back here, but I can't reach it, and the drawer is stuck."

The drawer was heavy and awkward, but after several tugs it slid out, empty. Frustrated, she got down on her knees and looked into the recesses. There was a dark, crumpled heap at the back of the drawer space. Reaching in, she grasped at a ribbon, gently tugged, and it popped loose.

It wasn't panties. She was holding a limp mass of sheer black organdy and purple-flowered gingham trimmed with a narrow band of purple ribbon. As she shook it out, she realized it was an apron. A child's bonnet, with a black organdy brim outlined in white lace and purple ribbon, formed a small pocket on the right side.

"Mama, what's an apron doing in your underwear drawer?"

As soon as she spoke, she regretted it. In the past two years of gradual, insidious memory loss, her mother had begun to squirrel away important items. It could be money, credit cards, or fine jewelry, and these episodes frequently created panic for the family and caregivers trying to find her forgotten hideaways.

Could the apron in the drawer be a part of Mama's paranoia? It's worth nothing, so why would she hide it in her underwear drawer?

"Oh, honey, I can't believe you found that. I wonder how long it's been there."

The aprons her mother wore were always kept in a kitchen drawer, directly below the one that held the dishrags and potholders. Most of them had pretty patterns with decorated pockets or some ornamental flair, including a few for holiday entertaining.

This one was of an entirely different genre. It was black, and the fabric was as transparent as tinted glass—not much help for wet hands or spills. The color and the lace on the pocket gave it a distinctly party aspect. The purple gingham flowers and the little bonnet pocket lent a paradoxical innocence to it. Feeling a slight weight on the side with the pocket, she reached in and withdrew a small, empty bottle with a ball-shaped pink cap. She could distinguish the words *White Shoulders Eau De Cologne* on the faded and worn label.

"Mama, did you know this was here? I've never seen it before."

"Oh, my goodness. It's been so long since . . ." Her mother's voice trailed off as she turned her gaze out the window.

"Mama, are you all right?"

She placed her hand tentatively on her mother's arm. It felt as fragile as the wing of a tiny bird. When her mother looked up, her eyes were damp. She reached into the waistband of her slacks, pulling out a worn white handkerchief with a tiny pink crocheted border and dabbed her eyes.

"I'm fine."

"It's all right, Mama. I lose things and then have happy accidental discoveries. Really. We all do it . . ."

"Honey, I forgot that it was in that drawer. I have *not* forgotten *why* it was there. And I'm not crying because it makes me sad. I'm just having . . . what do you call it, a little melting?"

"A little meltdown?"

"Yes, a little meltdown."

"Are you sure you're not upset? I don't want to bug you."

The memory challenges were a delicate subject.

"Should I put the apron back in the dresser, or in the kitchen with its cousins?"

She was trying to be funny, not sure where this was going.

"Just give it to me, honey. I'd like to hold it before we put it away."

Her gnarled fingers grasped the fabric. She laid it in her lap and began gently smoothing out the folds and wrinkles.

"Oh my, oh my," she chanted, mantra-like.

The daughter, mesmerized, realized she was still holding the little perfume bottle.

"Mama, this was in the pocket. It's empty. Should I throw it out?"

"Oh, no. Please, let me have it." She took the bottle, put it to her nostrils, then closed her eyes and inhaled deeply. "Mmm . . . I can still smell it."

With some effort, she awkwardly unscrewed the round pink cap and removed it. She leaned forward to the marble-topped table near her chair. It held a photo of her with her husband, dancing cheek to cheek at her eightieth birthday party.

She tapped the frame with the bottle.

"Can you smell it too, sweetheart? It looks like our little girl has discovered our secret."

She had a broad smile and a twinkle in her eye.

"I really haven't lost it, honey, though I'm sure you think I have. In fact, I don't think Daddy would care if I shared something special with you. You are an old married woman yourself now." She giggled.

"Gosh, Mama, do you really think I'm mature enough? After all, I'm *only* sixty-two."

"*That* old?" she quipped. "How did you grow up so fast?"

"Just like you, Mama. We blink and it happens."

"Well, this apron is probably almost as old as you are."

"Shouldn't it have more wear and tear with all that cooking and washing?"

"Oh, honey, it has never been in the kitchen." She paused, sighed, and softly stroked the apron as she resumed. "A long time ago when you kids were all little, your Daddy had to spend many hours at the hospital. Sometimes he wouldn't get home till after you were all tucked in and asleep. In those days it was impossible for us to find time or energy for those private moments all couples need. We were so busy, he with his work and I taking care of four children born in five and a half years. I was beginning to sense that I did not like what was happening to your Daddy and me. We were losing the romance that had first drawn us together. So, I bought a couple of what in those days were called marriage manuals. I hid them away because I did not want your Daddy to know I thought we might need help in *that* department. I'd read a chapter whenever I had a few spare minutes. Most of it was pretty mundane. I skipped a lot, looking for the parts about how to make our love life more—well, interesting."

She hesitated again.

"I can't believe I'm telling you this."

She giggled and the daughter noted the crescendo of animation in her mother's voice and facial expression. It was as though sixty years had magically dropped away from the small, frail body.

"You can't stop now, Mama."

"Well, the part of the book that really got my attention was the importance of good communication and planning, and also thinking about little things you could do to surprise your man. I thought and thought about what I could do that would be a really special surprise for your daddy. One day, I was shopping for a wedding gift downtown on Peachtree Street, and I went into Rich's Department Store. I started my search on the second floor in the kitchenware department, but I was distracted by a cooking demonstration at a small makeshift station. The female chef said, 'Ladies how would you like to cook up a little surprise for your husband tonight?'

"To this day, I don't know what it was she was preparing in that skillet, but I did notice she was wearing a skimpy black apron over her white uniform. I went up to her afterwards and asked her where she had gotten her apron. She pointed towards the pots and pans. I made a beeline and found stacks of pretty aprons. There were solid colors, pastels with flowers, stripes, plaids, polka dots, suns, stars, moons, bunny rabbits, ducks, roosters, sequins, bows, holly, poinsettias and Christmas trees, cows and pigs, eggs, bacon, and milk bottles. You name it—they had it. But I could not find anything even closely resembling the sheer black one the chef was wearing. I gave up. Then as I approached the escalator, the chef walked up to me and asked if I had found the apron I wanted. I told her no, everything but. She asked me if the apron I had in mind was a gift or was it just for me. I couldn't believe what I said next. 'It's a gift for my husband.'

"I think a light bulb switched on in her head because she asked me if I could wait a minute. She went back to her cooking area, took something out of a drawer, and put it into a bag. She was grinning like a Cheshire cat when she walked back over to me. She opened the bag, gave me a peek, and there was the black apron. She laughed and handed it to me. 'Have fun,' she said.

"You know, I can't tell you what I had for breakfast this morning, but I remember the ride down that escalator like it was yesterday.

"That night, Daddy asked me about my day. I told him I had watched a cooking demonstration at Rich's and that I would cook up a surprise for him very soon. He just nodded and said, 'That's nice.'

"The next weekend your grandparents wanted to take all four of you on a picnic at the Grant Park Zoo and then have you spend the night with them. I jumped on their offer like a cat on a June bug!

"Saturday, as Daddy was leaving for his golf game, he asked if I'd like to go out to dinner that night. I told him I thought a quiet evening at home would be nice."

She paused and took a sip of water from the glass on the table and smiled again at the photo.

"That afternoon, I fixed dinner and then took a long bubble bath. I curled my hair, did my makeup, and painted my fingernails and toenails. Then I put on the new apron over my black garter belt, black fishnet stockings, and my black, patent leather high heels. I added my black beaded necklace and matching earrings. That was it. Nothing else."

She was laughing.

"I was touching up my Revlon *Certainly Red* lipstick when I heard Daddy's car in the driveway. I grabbed the bottle of White Shoulders off the dresser and dabbed some behind my ears, on my temples, neck, wrists, and a little bit in my cleavage. That must have been when I slipped the bottle into the apron pocket. As soon as Daddy came through the door, I stepped out and said, 'Surprise!' He had a big smile on his face. 'Well, well, what's for dinner?' he asked. I said, 'The surprise I told you about. You're getting dessert *first* tonight.'

"I guess you don't need Paul Harvey to figure out the rest of the story, honey. This apron and the little bottle of White Shoulders lasted a long time, just like your Daddy and me."

The daughter watched her mother as she gathered the apron edges and carefully folded them, lining up the pocket on the outside and tucking the bottle of White Shoulders into it. She tenderly pressed the apron against her chest.

After a few moments of silence, she let out a long sigh. "The perfume is gone but the apron still has some wear left in it. Would you like to have it, honey? You found it and I'm so glad you did. It's yours if you want it."

"I'd love to have it someday, but not right now, Mama. You hang on to it for a little while longer. My finder's reward is the story."

The daughter felt herself blushing but couldn't stop from adding, "I'll bet when it came to cooking up surprises for Daddy, not even Betty Crocker could have competed with you and this magical apron of yours."

Suddenly animated again, her mother chuckled. "You know, your Daddy used to serenade me with his own off-key version of the Pillsbury jingle."

Her eyes flickered with mischief as she took a deep breath. Without missing a beat, she sang, "Nothin' says lovin' like somethin' from the oven . . ."

GOTCHA COVERED: A LEGACY OF SERVICE AND PROTECTION

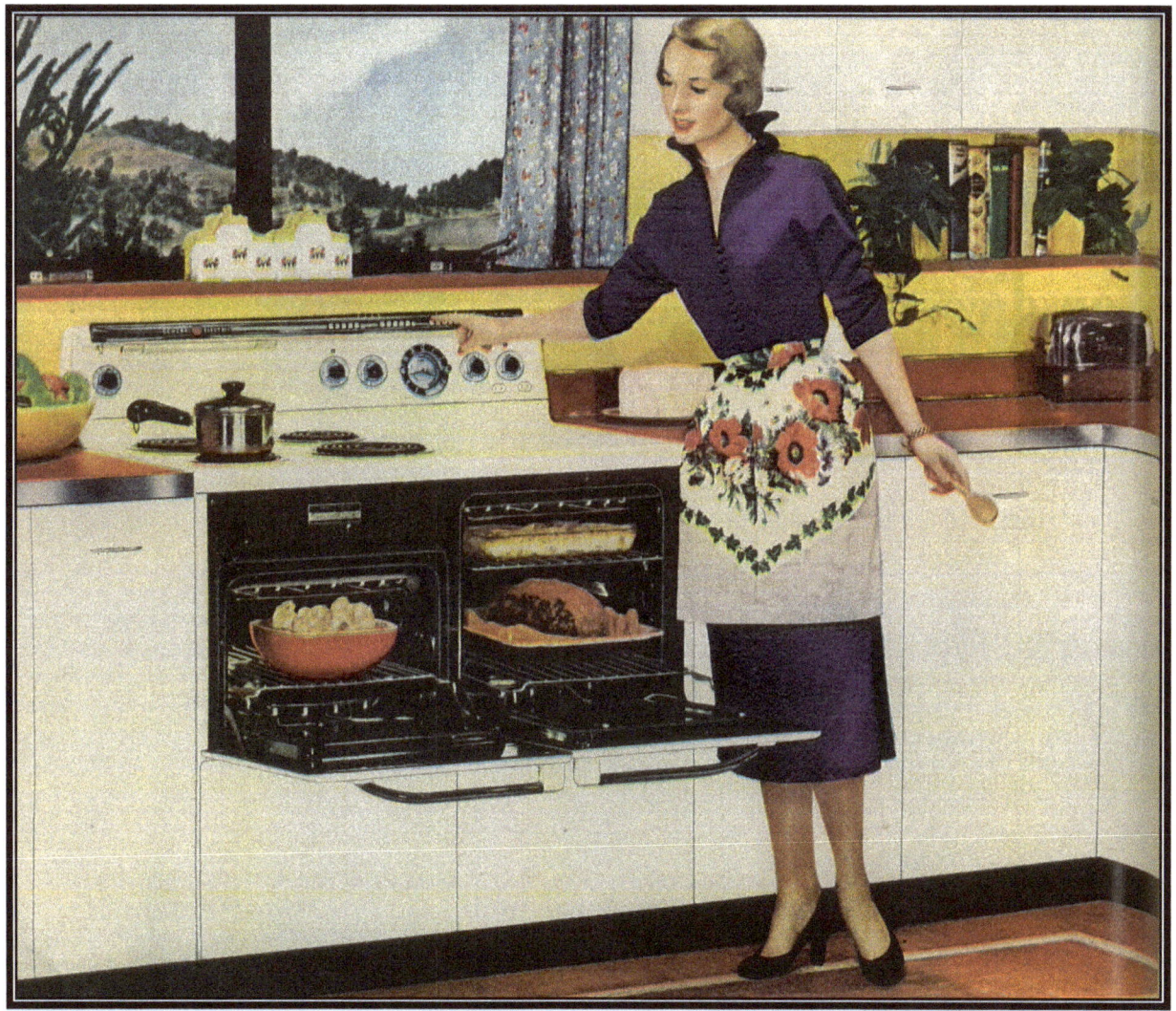

This G.E. ad for "huge master oven, companion oven" appeared in the March, 1952, *Better Homes and Gardens*, where it was one of eighteen images of apron-clad women shown in domestic venues in that issue of the magazine. © 1952 General Electric Company, used with permission.

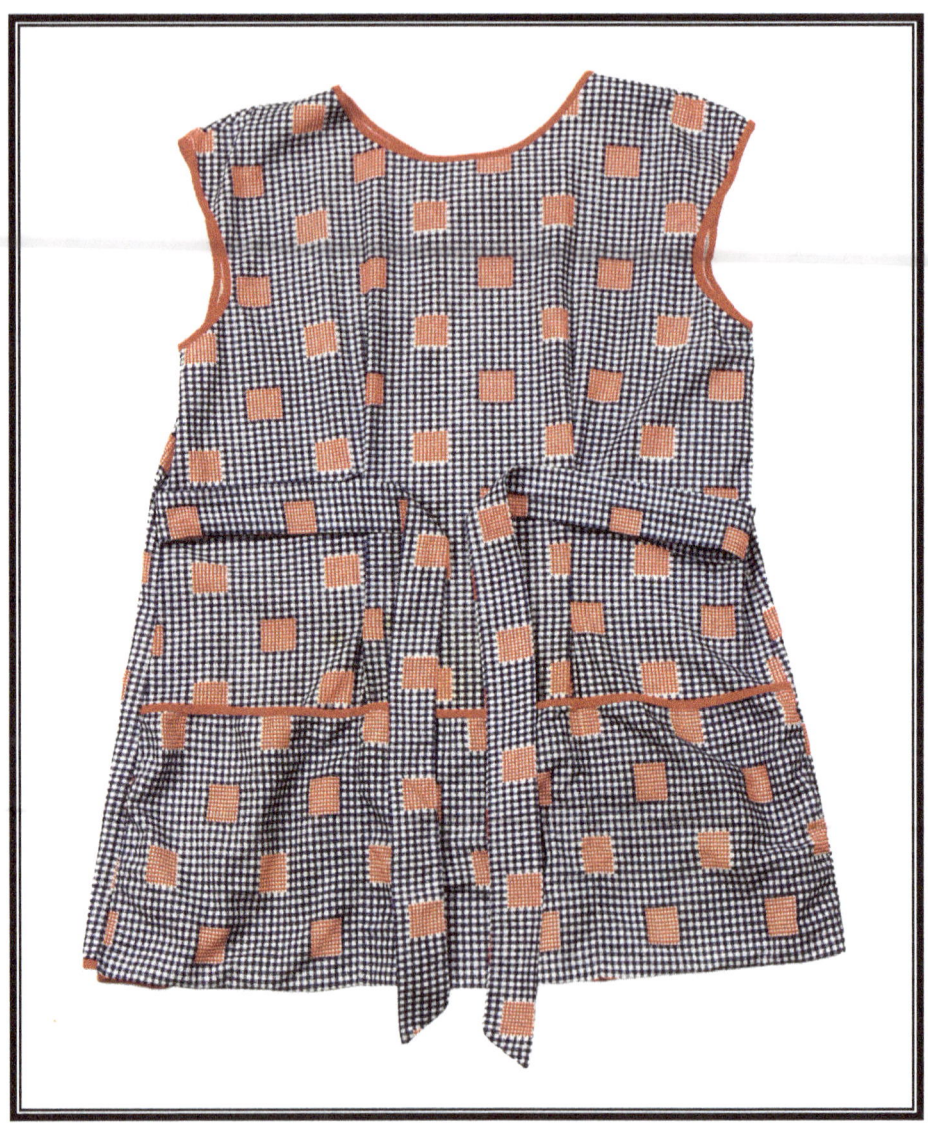

Adopted April 24, 2007 by Carol E. Dixon

The Worry Apron

Carol E. Dixon

I drag Patty's wheeled luggage to short-term parking, and she follows with her carry-on bag hooked over her shoulder. The minute we're in the car she starts bawling, and I bite my lip to keep from crying myself.

"I thought this was hard for me, but you're out of control, Sweet P," I say. "Let's stop for a little something on the way home and you can unwind, all right?"

My kid sister and I settle in a back booth at Young's Jersey Dairy with root beer floats jazzed up with chocolate syrup, the brown cows of our high school days. In five minutes I cover the preliminaries. The funeral for our grandmother, Beeble, had been simple. Mom and Dad had the wake at their house. Everybody understood Patty's airline snags and missing the funeral. Rumors were afoot that Aunt Rose had been going through our grandmother's house even before the funeral.

We finish our floats and spend the rest of the evening at my apartment in our pajamas, reminiscing over mugs of cocoa. Patty and I, in our twenties, are still chocolate addicts.

"Wish we had our Cinderella and Sleeping Beauty mugs now," Patty says.

"I don't remember what happened to them. This is Beeble's cocoa recipe though, marshmallows and all. Funny, Patty, I thought she was a rich woman because she gave us three marshmallows when she made our cocoa," I say.

"Me, I thought she was rich because she had that box of fancy buttons," Patty says.

When we were kids, our grandmother—whose name, Mabel, we'd mangled into "Beeble"—had a cookie tin full of majestic buttons—carved, painted glitters that we thought were real diamonds, nacre shells, gold anchors, filigreed silver—buttons as big as silver dollars and as tiny as our baby cousin's pinky fingernail.

"Nettie," she says to me with a wobble in her voice, "Beeble was poor and we didn't even know it."

"We were kids. How would we know who was rich and who was poor? She gave us our mugs and the button box to play with. She was rich."

The next morning, on the way to Beeble's house, I ask Patty if she's thought about what she'd like as a memento, *if* anything is left after Aunt Rose's raid. Aunt Rose is our Uncle Art's second wife—the one the family privately calls "Rustling Rose." She has a black dented pick-up that can't pass a garage sale or flea market, and her house has always looked like a junk shop. As kids, we'd get goose bumps at the mention of a trip to Uncle Art and Aunt Rose's house. She had shelves with bowling trophies, mustache mugs, zinc jar lids, hair lockets, sprung music boxes, old coins, ancient bed pans, nasal hair tweezers, a prosthetic leg, and a jar with two artificial eyes. Her weird medical gadgets were irresistibly frightening for Patty and me.

We're parked in the driveway by Beeble's side door when we notice Mister Baggins facedown in our grandmother's weedy backyard flowerbed. Patty and I gave her the gaudy plaster gnome when we were in grade school, and Beeble had pretended absolute astonishment. Setting Mister Baggins in the center of her prize tea roses, she declared, "My goodness, girls, I been waiting for a gnome for ever so long. I 'spect we won't have a bit of trouble with bears in the garden now, will we?" For years after that, Patty and I took complete credit for our grandmother's bear-free city neighborhood.

Now Patty points through the windshield at Mister Baggins' faded plaster Tyrolean hat and chipped lederhosen. "He looks so . . . so . . . decrepit, but he's still kind of cute," she says, putting on her "baby sister" face. "Can I have him, Nettie?"

"Sure, but you'll have to get him through airport security. They'll think he's loaded with drugs, of course." I laugh. "Anyway, I'm surprised Aunt Rose hasn't already swiped him."

Patty gives me her "you-didn't-say-that" look, and I apologize. "You're right, she's kind of strange, but she wouldn't take other people's stuff . . . would she? Patty, honestly, do you think Aunt Rose has been taking things from Beeble's house?"

"Who knows, Nettie? People get strange when it comes time to divvy up the family jewels—not that Beeble had any," Patty says. "The only jewelry I remember was her amber beads and the locket with the picture of her and Grandpa on their wedding day."

We step out of the car just as Aunt Rose's pick-up skids around the corner into the driveway and stops half an inch behind my bumper. She cranks down the driver's window, waves like a semaphore specialist, and yells in a deep, gravelly voice, "Girls, you just wait right there, hear?"

Aunt Rose galumphs around the back of her truck in unbuckled galoshes, black chinos, and a purple windbreaker inscribed, "Belmont Belles Bowling Champs."

"My gracious, girls, it's good to see you," she says, sidestepping me with a key ready to slip in the side door.

"How's Boulder, Patty?" Aunt Rose asks while she pushes past us into the kitchen and answers her own question. "Heard the Flatirons ain't much to see now with all the pollution, but I tell you girls, they was real pretty when your Uncle Arty and me was there for our honeymoon."

The kitchen is spit-spot, black enamel pots and pans hanging on pegs, the teakettle on a trivet by the stove, the toaster beside the knife rack on the counter. What I don't see is Beeble's black-and-white checked apron hanging on the hook by the fridge. And I don't see her pink Depression Ware cake plate in the corner hutch, or the milk glass hens sitting on their milk glass nests on the windowsill.

"Listen, girls, I got some things to take care of out in the garage. Think you can look around awhile, maybe give some thought to what you'd like? I'll be back 'fore you know it, all right?" Aunt Rose clomps out the side door.

Patty and I meander through the house noticing ordinary things iridescent with childhood memories: a dime store candy dish on the mantle, *Life* magazines on the end table, the barrister cabinet where Beeble kept the button box, the yellow wooden shoe she used for a door stop, a midnight-blue crystal vial on her dresser.

"It's just a perfume bottle, but I thought it was magic. Remember how she'd let us hold it and make a wish when we were good?" Patty asks.

I ignore her question, puzzling over an empty space on Beeble's dresser. "Patty, her jewelry box is gone."

We pull out drawers in her room, but there's no sign of her jewelry box.

"You looking for something, girls?" Aunt Rose says, suddenly standing in the doorway.

"Um, we're just wondering what happened to Beeble's jewelry box," Patty says.

"Oh, dear . . ." Aunt Rose starts.

"Seems like some other things are missing, too," Patty adds.

Aunt Rose reaches up her sleeve, pulls out a large white handkerchief and honks. "Sorry, girls, your grandma's garage is real dusty—a bad place for an old hen like me."

"Aunt Rose, what's going on?" I ask.

"Truth be told, girls, I wasn't supposed to say just yet. Your grandma wanted ever'body together when Arty told them how she wanted things. I 'spect the family's been noticing me around here a lot lately, probably wondering why, just like you're doing yourself, right? Fact is, I been trying to get things in order, the way your grandma liked." She goes on, "Well, ever'thing's here, honest and truly. Her special things are in the spare bedroom, like she asked."

Aunt Rose talks non-stop, leading us like a majordomo back to the kitchen. She opens a grocery bag and sets paper plates and napkins on the counter.

"Best set down, girls. This is not a short story, but it's true. I'll do my best to tell it like your grandma wished it to be told," she says, pulling out two kitchen chairs and shooing us toward the table.

"Your grandma and me been friends since me and your Uncle Arty got married. You might not know, but some in the family took exception to him marrying me so soon after your Aunt Stella died. Still, your grandma saw we was having a good life together, and she took me in like I was blood kin. Since then your grandma and me have had some whooping good laughs and some pitiful sad cries together.

"To me, she was right up there with the saints, nursing your grandpa all them years after his stroke and helping ever'body in the family *and* the neighbors to boot.

"This whole last year when me and Arty dropped by with her Sunday suppers, she'd set right here at this table pushing her hands deep down in her apron pockets till she near wore holes out the bottom. I think she fretted 'bout things, feeling bad she didn't have much to leave her children. It was real important what little mite she had should be shared fair and square."

Aunt Rose blows her nose again, washes her hands at the kitchen sink, and when she turns to look at Patty and me, her chin is quivering.

"She told how squabbling over things had near wrecked her own family when she was growing up, and I s'pose she didn't want to leave that kind of mess for her children. Said she was starting a list of ever' single thing she owned, adding new things at the bottom, scratching out what was gone, hoping to parcel things out even. Ever' Sunday night when me and Arty was ready to leave, she'd be working her hands down in the pockets of that old checked apron, still worrying over her list."

Aunt Rose looks down at the counter, waiting till she can get words out again.

"'Bout the time she got sick, that list kinda' wore out from all her fretting on it I 'spect. When her apron pocket was full of tatters, know what she said? 'Rose, I gave the best love I had to each one, and I gave them good memories. Now I'll have to trust they'll get through the sharing part without my parceling list when I'm gone.'"

Aunt Rose carries a tray to the table and says, "Your Uncle Arty will see to your grandma's wishes, just like he promised her, girls." Then she sets my old Cinderella mug in front of me and Patty's Sleeping Beauty mug in front of her, plopping three marshmallows into each one, pouring us hot cocoa from a thermos.

A week later at the airport, Mister Baggins has passed inspection and is on his way to Boulder.

"Nettie, thanks for letting me have him *and* the apron," Patty says.

"Hey, what good's a big sister if she can't spoil the baby in the family?" I say as she walks toward the "passengers only" corridor. I blow her a kiss and add, "Remember what Aunt Rose said. 'It don't do one bit of good carrying worries 'round in your apron pocket.'"

Gotcha Covered: A Legacy of Service and Protection

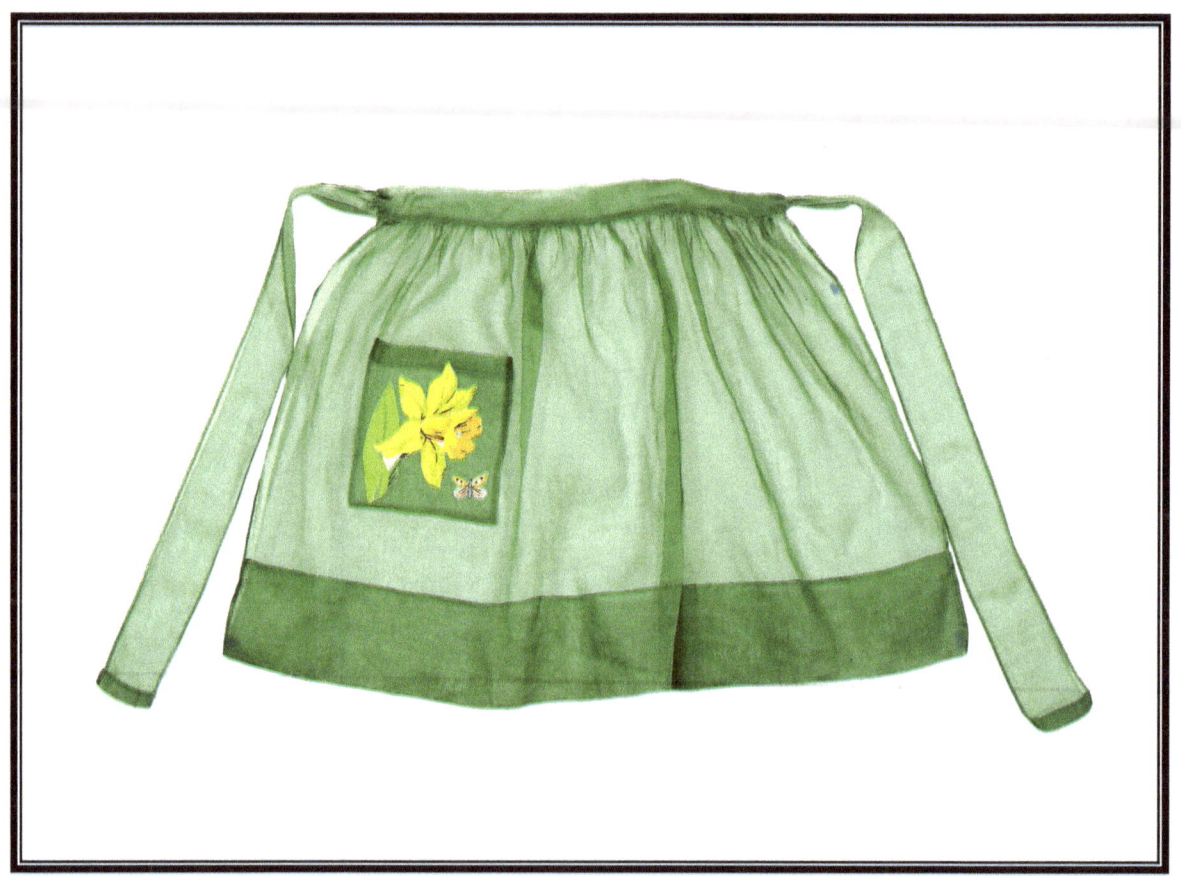

Adopted October 21, 2006 by Ellen E. McGeady

The Green Apron

Ellen E. McGeady

Leah sat alone in the cluttered little apartment, with half-filled boxes all over the floor and the furniture. Books had been taken off their shelves. CDs were scattered across the dressing table, and the closets stood open with naked hangers. The manager had asked her to clean out the apartment to make it ready for the next occupant following her mother's death. Leah had packed away the clothes and household items for the local shelter. Sorting through her mother's things was a painful task, but she had done it in the same way she had assumed the responsibility for her mother's care the last few years of her life—carefully and lovingly. It was the kind of job that the two of them should have been doing together, as they had done when Leah's father had died almost ten years ago. It seemed so strange not to be talking to her mother as she folded sweaters and gathered the various items together, so she talked to her anyway. Oh, she knew that her mother wasn't really there, but it felt comforting to talk as though she were helping with the task.

The beige shoes—her mother called them her "old lady shoes"—were packed away to send along with the pantsuits and other simple clothing. All her life, Leah remembered her mother wearing serviceable things. She had never evidenced any particular interest in what she wore, just that it should be practical.

In the far back of the closet, Leah found a box she had never seen before. The layer of dust dulling the original brown color, made it obvious it hadn't been opened for a very long time. Without giving it a second thought, she took off the lid and looked inside. Within, there was another slimmer box, white and rectangular in shape, and tied with what appeared to be a faded green satin ribbon. She pulled one end of the ribbon and lifted the lid. Tissue paper covered the contents, and a small white envelope peeped out from one of the sheets. She took the envelope, opened it, and read the contents.

Red,
Saw this at the railroad station and somehow it reminded me of our last beautiful evening together, don't ask me why. The color goes well with your hair, Red, and the flowers . . . well, you are lovely like the flowers to me. It was the only thing the damn railway station had, and I wanted to get you something before I left and somehow the time ran out. You know how that is. I'll think of you wearing this when I'm away.

There was no signature, and Leah was surprised to see an old-fashioned apron, gauzy and gossamer green, with yellow flowers. It was the kind of apron a hostess might have worn at a party sixty years ago, or so Leah thought. It was certainly not anything her mother would have worn.

But who had written the note? The handwriting was not her father's, and Leah sensed that what she was looking at represented an aspect of her mother, totally unknown and mysterious. It was as if, in reading this note and seeing this apron, Leah became aware of the possibility of a whole new dimension of her mother. How odd that Leah had spent so many hours with her and not known anything about the author of this note. She didn't know when it was written, what it meant, who the person was—nothing—only the fact of it, and the green apron with the beautiful yellow flowers.

Who was this person? Was he a boyfriend? Where was he going? Where was Dad in all this? Her head filled with scattered thoughts and questions. She removed the apron and looked underneath. Tied together neatly, was a very small stack of letters. There were no dates, but the handwriting was the same as on the white card. Leah opened the first letter and began reading.

Dear Red,

I've had a really hard time of it since I got here. Every day we've been operating on our boys fighting in the Pacific. I feel like I'm knee deep in blood sometimes. The nurses have been wonderful, keeping us well supplied with coffee, but I told mine that all it was doing was giving me the shakes.

I got your last letter and I can't tell you how much it meant to me. Just knowing that there is someone at home that tells me I matter, makes me feel alive. Each day is worse than the last and there is no end in sight. Can't tell you where we are, but it's close to where some of the action is going on.

I miss our tennis games and good Scotch. Have to do that when I get back. Hope the children aren't having too bad of a time of it, what with all the shortages. Got to get some sleep. Hope to hear from you again soon.

It was signed, "David." That was not her father's name, and this would have been at a time when Leah's parents were already married. How had she been able to keep this a secret for so long? How had Leah not known even the existence of this David? She and her mother talked every day, and in all the years of conversations, this had never been brought up. It mattered to Leah that something had been withheld from her, when she had thought they had shared everything.

The next letter seemed grimmer.

Dear Red,

The war continues at an unrelenting pace. We are operating day and night. Sometimes I forget how long I've been in the tents, and when I do get a chance to walk outside, it's already the afternoon of the next day. There is no privacy and hot showers are non-existent. Sometimes the noise, the smell, and the constant dying make me feel like I'm going to go mad. Your letters are the only things that keep me sane. I can't wait for the day when I return and we can sit and read poetry together, or walk in the warm sunshine of an autumn day. Did that time before the war ever exist? My brother wrote that my mother has had a mild stroke. I can't worry about it now, even though I do. They're calling me. Must go. Write soon.

David

Not "love, David", but just "David" Was this an affair or not? *I wish it were,* Leah realized.

Dear Red,
 Your letter came today and it was all I could do not to get up and just run out of the tent to read it. You needn't worry about James; he'll find himself in time. He's a good boy and I'm sure he'll settle down, and you're a good mother, so not to worry. There's nothing you can do for my mother at this point. Thank you for asking. She's doing quite well, Henry tells me. I told her that you were a dear friend and that you might call. I can't tell you
 where I am, though it doesn't really matter much. Death and destruction is all there is. I was thinking about the parties you had at your house, don't ask me why. You were such a great hostess. Always made everyone feel comfortable and welcome, including yours truly. I'm such a dud at things like that. I just stand around. I've been humming that beautiful sextet from Lucia di Lammermoor. *You know the one. That's what we'll have to do when I get back—go to the opera. I miss our afternoons playing piano or listening to the phonograph. I think of you when I think of music. I wish this war would end.*

David

Dear Red,
 Sometimes it happens that people experience a connection through music. I grant you that. So you went with Carol to the opera without me. I'm jealous, but delighted that you got an opportunity to get out of the house. No green aprons for you, just sensible white ones. What a pity Stan cares so little for classical music. Thanks for the package of books, they arrived a week ago. I wish I had time to read them, but the life of a surgeon in war pretty much precludes the possibility. But I'll try, I promise. Which one should I read first? Which was your favorite? I'll try and guess. It's the anthology of poetry, isn't it? I like Robert Browning's, "Grow old along with me, the best is yet to be" or something like that. I think he means well and it's beautifully written, but it's not true you know. Growing old without the people you love is simply terrible. I think about that a great deal since I've been here. Most of these boys won't grow old at all. And they are just boys, Red. That I can tell you. We're all afraid that our time will run out and that we won't have done the things we dreamt of doing. Our possibilities will be over. The worst sound in the world is listening to a grown man crying for his mother. It haunts me in my sleep. I will hear it forever.

David

The letters were almost gone, and Leah knew somehow the outcome could not be good.

Dear Red,

They are moving us closer to the front so that we can give the boys our help more quickly. I don't know when I'll have the chance to write again. If for some reason you don't hear from me, you can always contact my brother, Henry, or my mother. I'll be thinking of you in any spare moments I have. I wanted to be here helping the war effort in any way that I could, and this is all I know how to do. I didn't know I would feel this alone, even when I'm surrounded by hundreds of people. I didn't know how much I would miss you. I keep thinking of the first time I met you. Remember? It was at the concert. You came alone, as I did, and we bumped heads when I stooped to pick up the program you had dropped. You started laughing and then I laughed, and before I knew it we were talking like old friends. I'll never forget how lovely I thought you looked wearing that green dress that brought out your red hair. I only had eyes for you, Red. You did know that, didn't you? I hope your family appreciates you. You should be appreciated. You're such a great lady. I don't know what the future will bring. I don't even know if there will be a future, but if I have a future then I want to be a part of yours, if I can. I know I have no right to write to you and say these things, but the war takes away many of our inhibitions, what with all the pain that is around us. When I see you Red, I hope we can start again where we left off. Please think about it before you say anything. I've weighed it as best I can and I've tried to be dispassionate, but of course I can't. You must know that by now.

Yours, David

The rest of the box contained a headline from a yellowed newspaper that screamed the latest casualties from Guadalcanal. Leah did not try to find the name in the column. She folded the paper, retied the few letters, and studied an old photograph of her mother standing next to a man wearing an Army uniform. Leah had never seen him before. Her mother looked so radiantly happy standing there with him. Leah had seen her mother in moments of joy, but she had never seen the look that was on her mother's face in that picture. What it must have cost her all these years to have kept this love a secret. How little we really know of one another.

He must have been killed; and what had her mother felt? She had saved all these things for so many years—the apron, the letters, the picture. Did she ever look at them again, in some quiet and secluded moment?

I'll never know, Leah thought, *but I hope that she had some beautiful moments with him, and I hope she didn't resent us, because we loved her too. She was our mother. We didn't think of her as a woman with all the yearnings and desires of women. We thought of her simply as our Mom. Our Mom wore sensible shoes and sensible clothes, and we never saw her in green, gauzy aprons with yellow flowers, but I'm so glad someone did.*

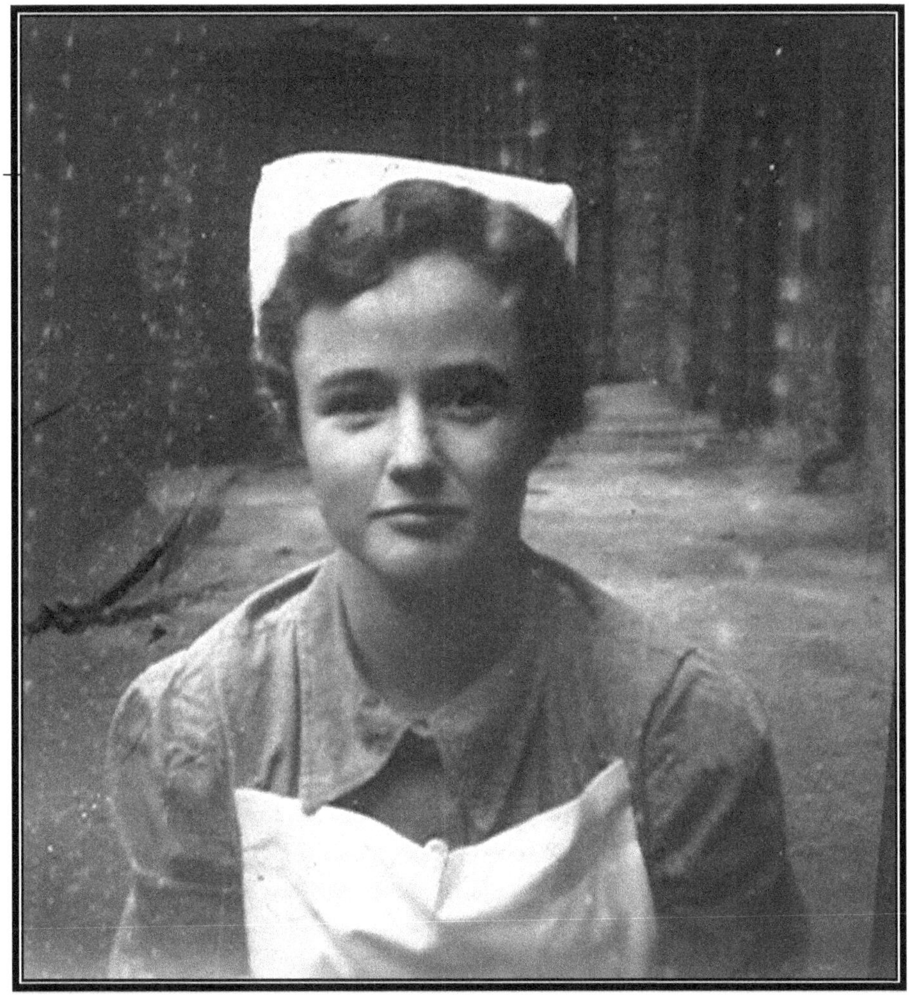

GOTCHA COVERED: A LEGACY OF SERVICE AND PROTECTION

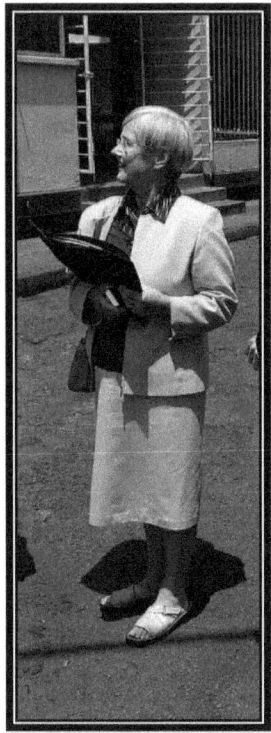

Eileen Richardson shown in her student uniform with apron, c.1956 at the Royal Infirmary of Edinburgh.

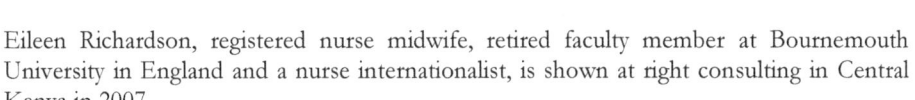

Eileen Richardson, registered nurse midwife, retired faculty member at Bournemouth University in England and a nurse internationalist, is shown at right consulting in Central Kenya in 2007.

GOTCHA COVERED: A LEGACY OF SERVICE AND PROTECTION

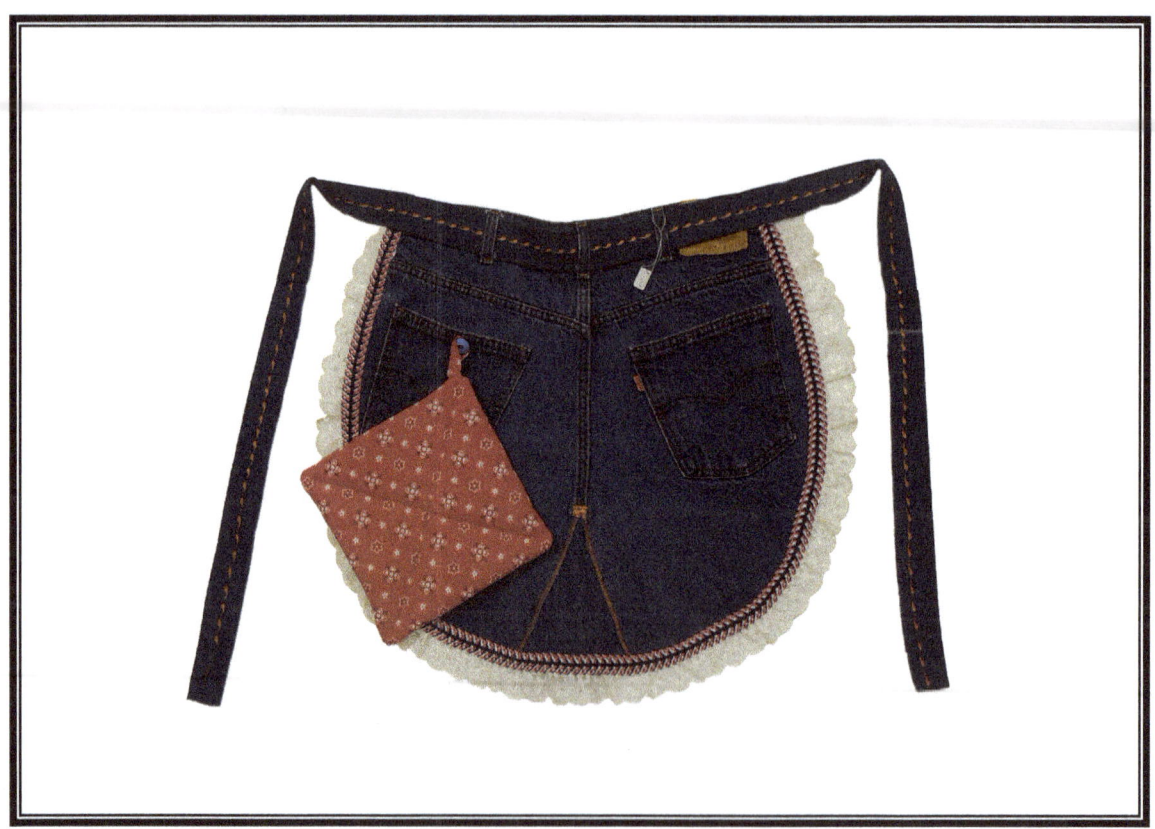

Adopted November 15, 2006 by Judy Tincher Monaco

Montana Memories

Judy Tincher Monaco

Look at me; I am filled with stains from many a meal prepared out in the windswept prairie grasses of Montana or in the foothills of our majestic mountains. You see, I have been worn on yearly cattle drives from the family homestead in the Paradise Valley up into the majestic Absaroka Mountains, when my family would drive the cattle into their leased summer grazing fields each June.

I was made by hand six generations ago in the early 1900s, when Montana was a new state. There was no electricity, health care, or highways. Just sooty oil lamps, herbs and potions, and ruts and animal paths among the grasses. Each member of our family relied on the benevolence of the weather, the care of other homesteading families, food raised in our kitchen gardens during our short, hot, and often dry summers, and a strong faith in God to protect us in this wild, harsh environment.

Each June, I would be folded up and placed near the portable cook stove of the head cattleman's wife, and brought out twice each day during the preparation of breakfast and dinner. You may wonder why there is lace around my hem. Life was hard, and no woman ever wore a pretty dress other than on her days of marriage and burial. She worked beside the men to make the ranch successful. This lace was torn from the hem of a party dress brought from back east and served as a reminder of a far easier life the wife could only dream of.

Life as I have described it has not changed much over the years. My present owner still helps with the annual cattle drive along with neighbors. Of course, there is now the Internet to stay in touch during the long, windy, grey winters. Grocery stores thirty minutes away and excellent health care. However, the basic values of my owner today are still the same: a strong work ethic, an abiding faith in God to moderate the weather, and a wonderful sense of humor to sustain her during hard times.

Gotcha Covered: A Legacy of Service and Protection

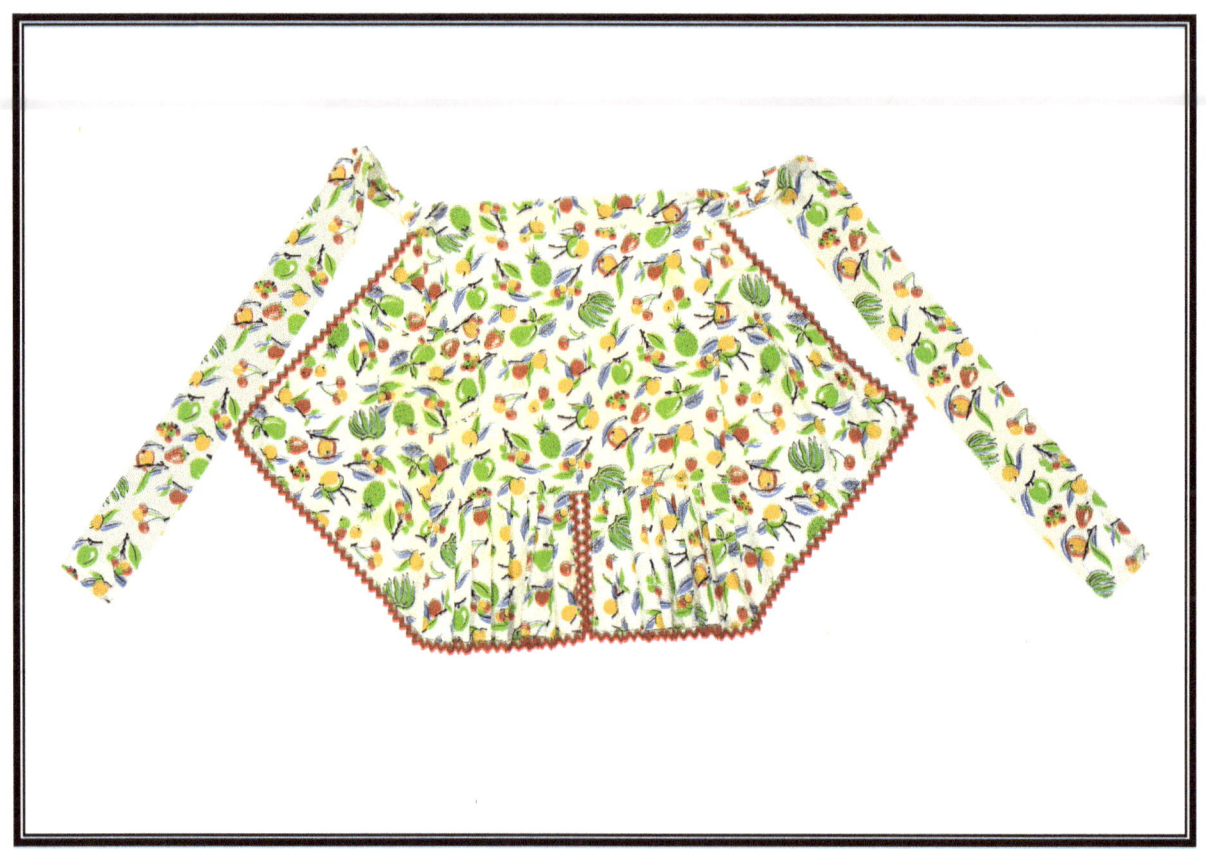

Adopted December 10, 2006 by Frances McGaughy Edwards

The Remnant

Frances McGaughy Edwards

I began as a remnant. I belonged to a bolt of fabric that someone bought for curtains. I am what was left, so I ended up on the remnant table. I saw the store owner's wife picking through the remnants all around me. She would pick up each one and feel it. I think she was trying to decide what she could make out of each one. She picked me up, checked the measurements, felt the fabric, and carried me to the cash register. I was overjoyed that someone wanted me. Now, my worry was, what will she make? I did not have long to wait for this lady, named Frances, to begin to cut out an apron. Now I was to be no ordinary apron. I was a fancy one with seven pleats on each side and a split in the middle. To go with all the cherries and strawberries on me, she added red rickrack all around the edge. So here I am, a classy apron, with all my fruit on the white background, pleats, and red rickrack. Oh, joy!

I had been in the apron drawer for only a few days before the cook, Alma, discovered me. Each morning, Alma came at seven o'clock and cooked breakfast for the family. She always checked the news in the paper and then listened to the news on the radio. I'd be tied around her middle, trying to understand what this was all about. The news was seldom happy. Except for the weather, it was always about a conflict of some sort. When the family came for breakfast, Alma always announced the horrors she had heard with this statement—"Folks can get themselves in some of the awfulest messes." Alma was very afraid of storms. Whenever the clouds would gather, she would look out the window and say, "Those are viggrus clouds over there." I could feel her fear and stayed close.

Alma was an excellent cook, even though she vowed and declared that she hated to cook. As sons-in-law began to arrive in the family circle, she would really show off for them, of course with me around her middle. She would cook mustard greens, corn bread, and have tomatoes and onions for making "Mr. Norton's" mixed-up dinners, and congealed salads; the girls called it a "shaky salad." Miss Frances would bring home new recipes, and she and Alma would make them. Miss Frances loved to cook, so she had my happy self tied around her middle most often. I remember the day she got her Mixmaster. It was at the end of World War II, and the advertisement in the paper for this new gadget was offered on a first-come-first-served basis. Well, she got up early and headed for the hardware store to buy one. Several hours later, she triumphantly brought this thing home. She tied me around her waist and went to work. First, she made a white cake, then the caramel icing. She and Alma could not contain their amazement that this machine could beat the cake batter and then the icing with so little effort. Now all of us were happy. One of the daughters came home after she had married, tied me around her middle, and taught Alma and Miss Frances how to make homemade mayonnaise with this machine. Miss Frances and Alma continued to use this wonderful gadget until they stopped cooking altogether.

Every time I was washed, Alma would carefully iron me and all my rickrack. She would not let anyone wear me for several days. I think she just liked to admire me and her ironing for a while. She was never happy if one of the girls or Miss Frances grabbed me off the ironing board and tied me around her middle. You see, I was the favorite apron in the house.

I lived in the apron drawer for many years, being washed, ironed, and keeping someone from getting food preparation on her clothes. Alma and Miss Frances made sure I was always without stains. One day, Alma did not come anymore. I wondered what had happened to her, then I heard Miss Frances say she had retired. The family began to leave home; one to nursing school, one to study English, and one to study business. Then Mr. Norton died one May evening, and all the families came home. Several years after that, Miss Frances decided it was time to close her house and move, and she began to give things away. When she came to the apron drawer, she gave me to her daughter, Frances.

She loves to cook, as do her daughters and her now-retired husband, Bill. I am used often (but not by Bill, yet). I've gained some stains here and there, but when I'm washed and ironed, who can tell with the jumble of pineapples, bananas, cherries, apricots, and strawberries on me? When this Frances decides to move, I wonder which daughter or daughter-in-law will want me. I hope I will be passed to someone else who will love me and include me in her family life.

NONFICTION

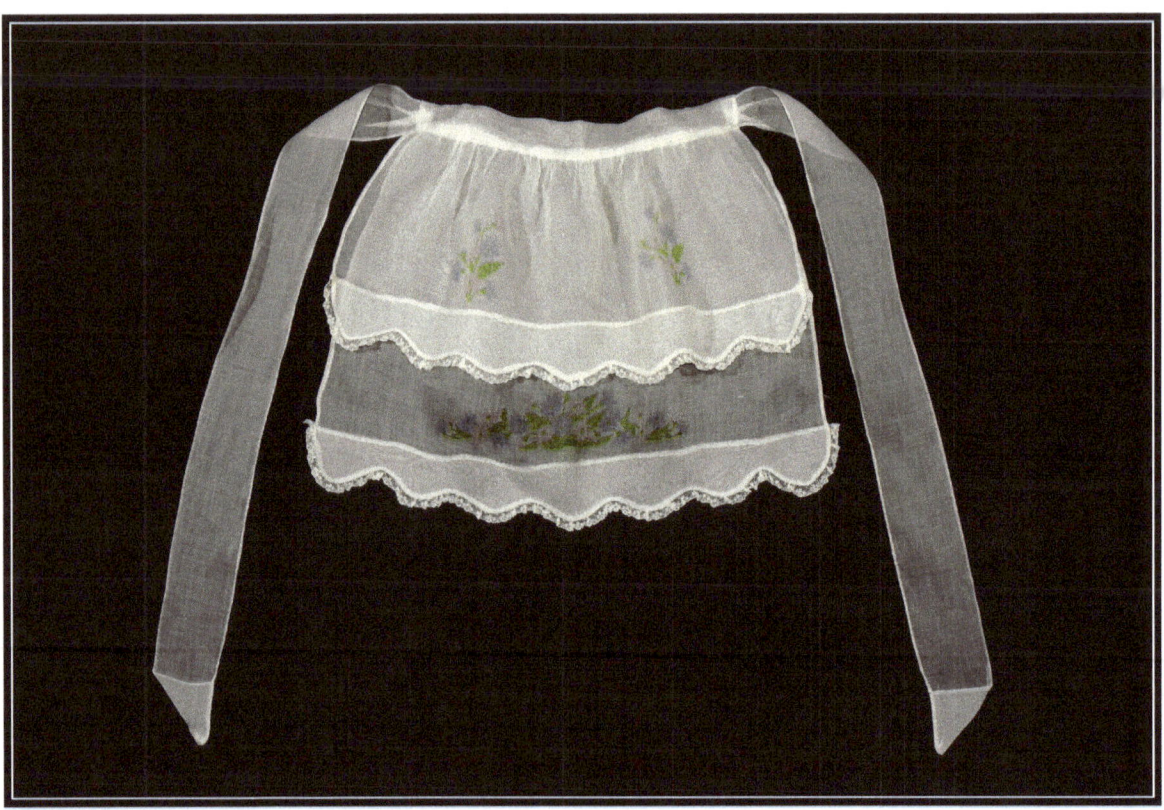

Adopted March 23, 2007 by Lydia Luttrell Grubb

The Wedding Apron

Lydia Luttrell Grubb

The tale of the wedding apron was just family lore that had never been verified. My mother told me, her mother told her, and so on. The story went like this:

Many years ago, my great-grandmother was slipping off to the woods to enjoy nature, or so her family believed. Eventually, it was discovered that Lydia was, in fact, visiting a dressmaker who was making a wedding gown, and other odds and ends for her elopement. She had been forbidden to see the young man she loved. His family was of lowly means and maintained questionable behavior throughout the community.

After the entire plot was discovered and stopped, my great-grandmother eventually married the family's choice for her husband. Some said she only tolerated him, as he publicly showed his adoration with slobbery kisses on her face and lips. She was a dutiful daughter, wife, and mother of three until she died at the very early age of twenty-six. The death certificate read "tuberculosis," but many believed that her death was caused by a broken heart.

Of course, my mother and I knew her only through this fragmented story. There were two other pieces of the story that have also been passed down through the years. One is that despite having a few fine pieces of jewelry, it was an apron that she treasured all her adult life. No one knew why, but everyone knew to keep it safe, protected, and special, out of respect and in honor of her.

I was looking at aprons in a craft shop the other day when I spotted an apron, which was similar and reminded me of my great-grandmother's apron. I asked the proprietress the significance of the pattern, and she stated it had always been called "the wedding apron." That prompted me to go home and rummage around to find Grandmother's apron, and to show more care for it than I had previously done.

When I located it, I was ashamed of the yellowed, wrinkled condition of her treasured apron. I resolved to work very carefully with it and make it white, crisp, and beautiful once more. I would display it in a shadow box or in some other creative way. If it meant so much to my great-grandmother, I would continue to make it special.

I researched gentle washing procedures, soaps, and whitening agents, but I was told that nature's whitening—the sun—was the safest. After carefully hand washing it, I took the apron outside to dry in the hot sun. When I returned to get the dried apron, I was dismayed to see that a black substance oozed all around it. The sun also reflected flashes of tiny, bright flecks around the fabric. Moaning, I grabbed it to investigate. It was tar! Upon further checking, I was amazed to find that a fine thread, woven into the material, was actually a very thin gold chain, which had been coated with a layer of tar and then a white coating to conceal its shiny worth.

I desperately needed to work on the tar and to decide what to do with the precious gold thread chain, but I also needed to know more about this apron and my great-grandmother's strong protectiveness of it. I visited the community where Grandmother Lydia had been reared, looked in old records and archives, and found the name of the dressmaker and read about her. A contemporary of Lydia's, and also a victim of the War Between the States, she was a master of concealing jewelry in clothing. That was really what she was more famous for than her dressmaking ability.

I still did not know the answer to the question of where my great-grandmother had gotten the gold chain. I will probably never know all the facts about this apron, but I have done a lot of fantasizing and embellishing of the few facts I have. Here is my take on the chain, apron, and my great-grandmother.

I have seen pictures of my great-grandmother's wedding dress—the one meant for her elopement, but actually worn in her wedding. Through the years, my great-grandmother was wearing her apron in many old family pictures with her children and family. I think that the dressmaker made the apron out of pieces of her wedding dress and, upon seeing how heartbroken my great-grandmother was about the change in her engagement, she offered to conceal something special to keep with her always. Grandmother Lydia chose a necklace. I suspect that the man she really loved gave her a gold chain necklace to wear around her neck, under her clothing, where it was unnoticed by the family. So, my great-grandmother always had a part of her beloved relationship literally around her, when she wore and treasured the apron.

I now smile and wonder if the part of my great-grandmother's life that I have surmised has the same basis of truth as the part of her life that was handed down to me. Have different generations passed tidbits sprinkled with truths and romance through the years?

The last little snippet of the story that I did not imagine, but that has always been shared and passed along with the aborted-marriage story, is that Grandmother Lydia's lost love vowed to better himself. He became educated. He never married. He became the governor of my great-grandmother's home state.

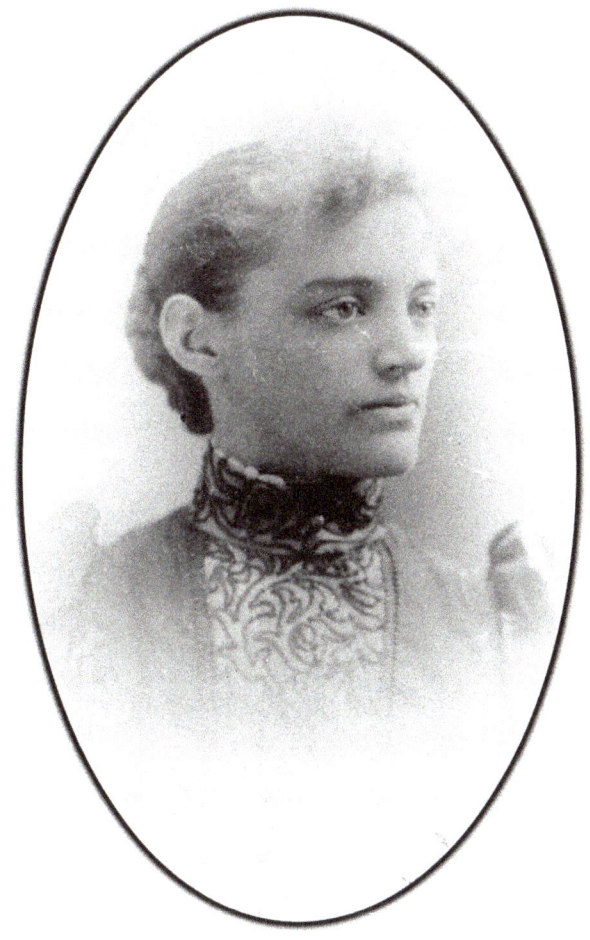

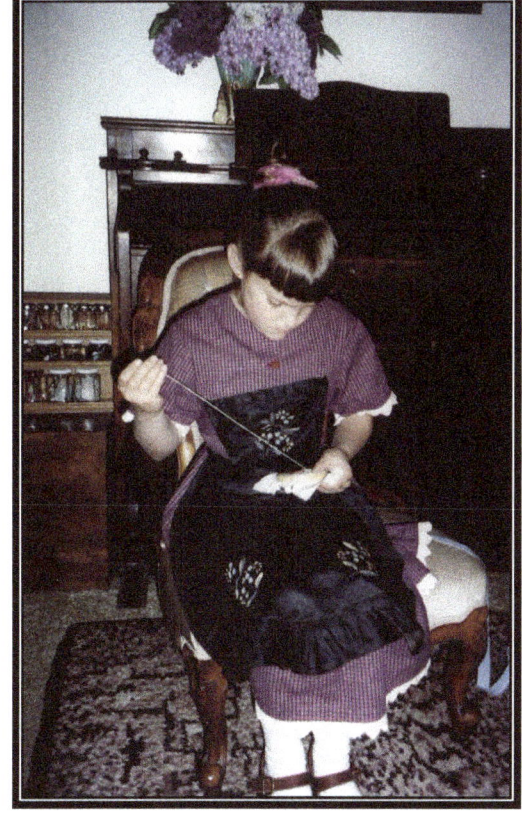

Lydia Grubb's great-grandmother, Lydia Richardson c.1890. No photographs of Grandmother Lydia in her wedding apron were available. Photo submitted by Lydia Grubb.

Michaela Smith, granddaughter of Avis Smith, at age 8 (c.1998) wearing an 1880's child's parlour apron on which are embroidered forget-me-nots. In 2009, Michaela is pursuing her Bachelor in Nursing degree as a first year student at the University of Adelaide. Photo submitted by Avis Smith.

Gotcha Covered: A Legacy of Service and Protection

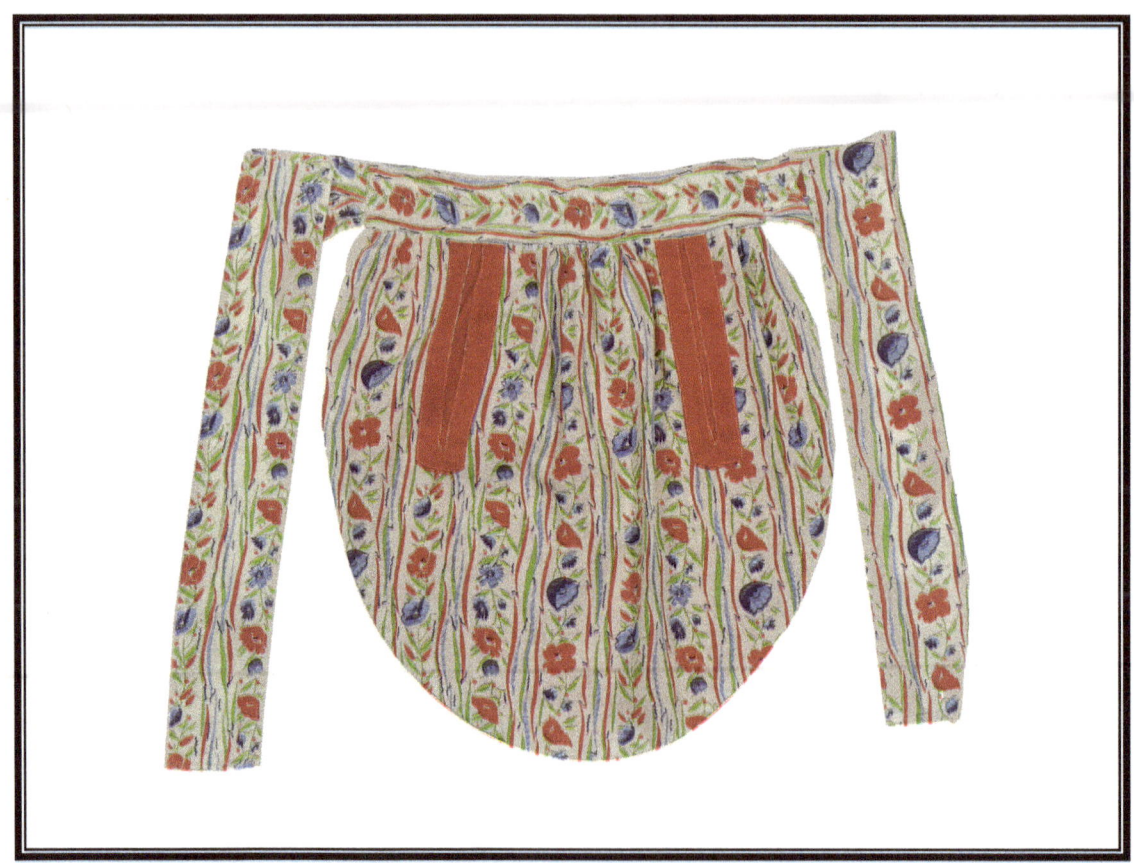

Adopted December 1, 2006 by Myra Wilson Willey

A Pocket Surprise

Myra Wilson Willey

She lived down the street behind a brick wall.
We secretly watched as she gardened there.
My sister and I were a little afraid—of what I don't know.
She never did anything to give us a scare.

Tall and slender and dignified, she
Would work quietly as we sat on her wall.
We never thought she would see us there,
Until the day she beckoned us with a call.

From that day on we often returned
To visit her in that garden or home.
She told us good stories and showed us her treasures,
But the best was yet to come.

When we finished a visit and were ready to go,
She would walk us to the gate so far.
She'd reach into her deep apron pocket
And give each of us a chocolate bar.

We finally grew older and we visited no more.
But we never forgot that sweet lady,
Who took time for two girls with her lore,
And the surprise in the deep-pocketed apron she wore.

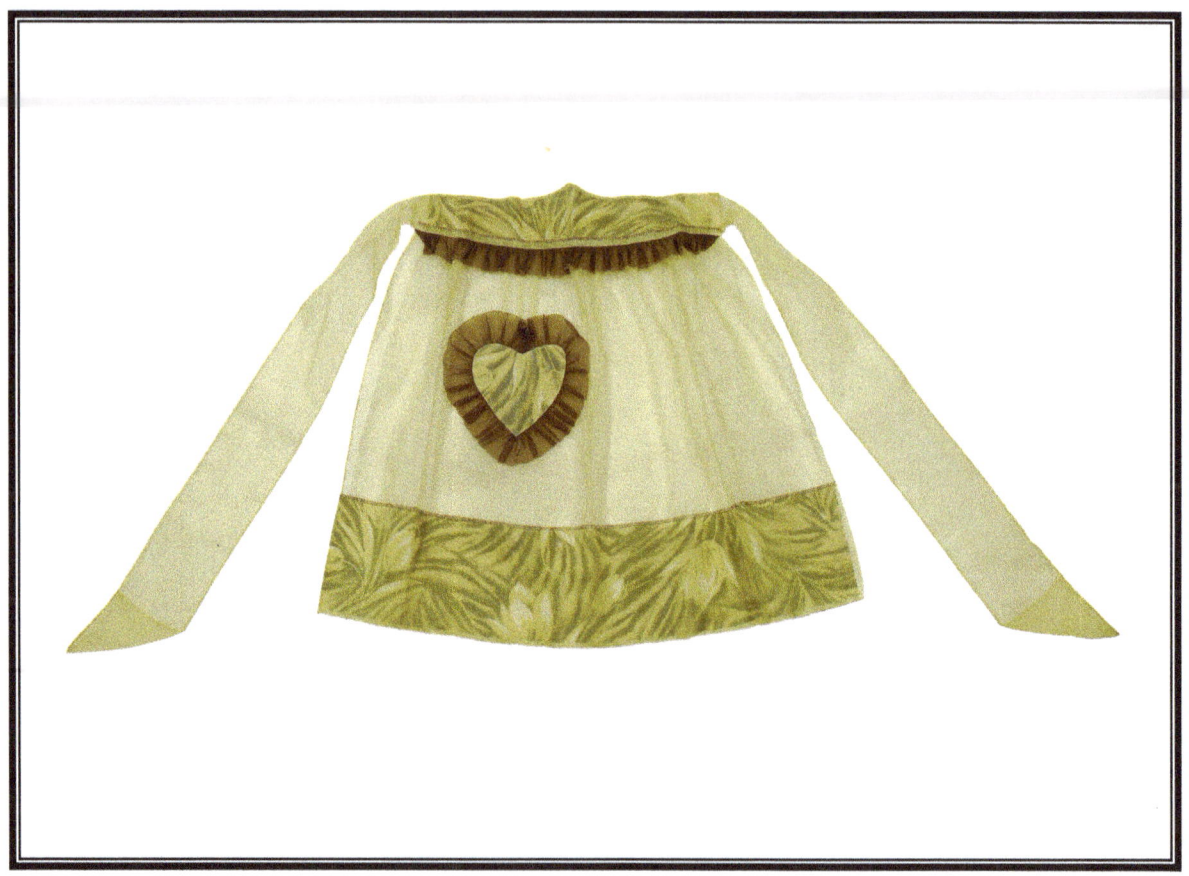

Adopted February 1, 2007 by Louise Colln

Louise Colln submitted a transcription of an interview, done with a woman she knew who lived in rural Missouri.

The Happy Childhood of Grandma Ida Gilmore

Louise Colln

I was born in what they call Ozark County, in Missouri. I was the third child, and there were eleven of us when I got married, but we ended up with fifteen, so that was quite a family. My parents were John and Frances Rowland. They were born in Missouri, but their parents came from Tennessee. I really wasn't interested in the past so much till in my later years, and I found there wasn't anybody to ask about a lot of things.

My mother had the best memory. But when I asked her about our ancestors, she didn't know too much about it. They all came to Taney County, Missouri, in wagons, sometime in the 1800s.

My mother's father was Henry Simpson, and my other grandfather, I believe his name was John. I heard my mother say that he didn't want to be called "Grandpa" and that made me kind of shy with him. I just kind of slipped around and stayed afar. Of course, there was so many of us he didn't miss me.

They didn't live close. They came and visited us a time or two. He and my uncle had two wagons and they stayed awhile. They just kind of traveled. I guess kind of gypsy-like. They'd stop and work, and then they'd travel on.

We left Ozark County, though, and went to a little town called Gritty. We went to school at what's called "Truevine." Then we moved to Bradleyville. At that time, we went by horse and wagon, and I imagine it seemed like a lot of miles, where it wouldn't seem so far now. Then we lived close to Forsyth. That was the old town. The one that went under the waters. Even the courthouse. It was down in the bottom. They just tore it away, though, and built the new one on the hill. We lived between Forsyth and Taneyville, and it was hilly. It was always just a common house. We never did have a house that was big enough for the family, but we managed.

We had a bed-full when we slept. Upstairs, downstairs. It was nothing for three or four to sleep in one bed. Kept us warm. Sometimes we kept things like our potatoes for the winter under the bed, because we had to keep them from freezing. We went to a one-room school. And we carried water from a spring and all drank out of the same dipper. Took our lunch in little buckets or whatever. And we played baseball, but our bat was a board trimmed down so we could get our hands around it. We didn't have much to do with.

We had to get up early in the morning, but we didn't have a whole lot of chores to do before we went to school. We just had a few cows to milk. We wasn't selling milk then. We had a few chickens to have eggs, and usually just a few hogs to have our own meat.

We went nut hunting in the fall—walnuts and big hickory nuts and a few hazelnuts. They used to burn over the fields, and where they did, the hazelnuts was killed out. We'd go out to wild blackberries patches in fields and fencerows. I didn't enjoy picking blackberries. But I did it because I had to.

None of us older kids learned to swim. Mama was so afraid of water. She just wouldn't let us in water for fear we'd get drowned. Half of us could have got drowned and she'd have plenty left, but she didn't think so. And since I couldn't swim myself, I didn't want my children to go in the water either. I didn't have any children to spare.

When we were growing up, we made our own clothes. We didn't know what bought clothes were. And we wore them till they was all worn out. My mother did most of the sewing at home because she was pregnant so much of the time, and she could sew when she couldn't do other things. It took a lot of sewing with that many children. But she would start in the early spring making us clothes and getting us ready.

A month or two ahead of time anyhow, for they most always had a Fourth of July picnic. They'd pick out a wooded area on the edge of town where they had cleaned it out. That was when I got to eat bananas. And lemonade. Mama would cook and take lunch for us, and we'd spread the tables. But sometimes we would buy lemonade. I believe they sold hamburgers, but I didn't get any. They probably cost too much. We couldn't afford it with all the bunch. That would be a lot of hamburgers for sure. Mama would get with others that was like she was, always nursing a baby and little ones all around. They'd take chairs so she could sit down and a quilt for the kids. Pallets, they called them, for the little kids to waller on and sleep and so forth.

It seems to me like we would have a play at school before Christmas. A Christmas play. We just got candy at Christmas. We never thought about presents. We didn't know what they was.

I remember going to Grandpa Simpson's at one time and Santa Claus just left a good big sack of mixed candy on the stairs, and somebody passed it around and we all had candy. That was a big treat. We enjoyed it just as much as we do now because it was a day to get together with people.

I used to have a playhouse. I'd lay rocks around to divide the rooms, and then use broken dishes. I'd always save what got broken in the house. I was just as happy as if I'd had bought stuff. It was always under a tree, and I'd pick berries or something like that, and take mud and make pies and just had the most fun.

Back when I was growing up, our way of going was horseback a lot. I had an older brother and sister, and we three would all go to pie suppers and dances together. I had to ride behind with my sister. She was older, so she got the saddle.

The pie suppers was to make money to do something for the school. You made a pretty box and put the pie in it, and they would be sold by auction. And the boys would try to buy their girl's pie. They weren't supposed to know whose pie it was, but they usually found out. Then, when they were all sold, why, you'd sit down and eat the pie together.

The fun part was decorating the box. Oh, it was the prettiest box. You have no idea how much crepe paper was used. We'd take boxes and round them, put a handle on them and just decorate them all up with crepe paper to make them look pretty.

We had square dances too. We'd empty out the back bedroom and have square dances in it. We'd get somebody to play the music. I remember one time all we had was a fiddle to dance by, but it was the best music. We just had the most fun you wouldn't believe.

* * *

Ida met her husband, Dee, at a pie supper when she was sixteen. Over the years, they worked modern, successful farms together, and reared two children. Her grandson remembers going out early to feed and care for the animals, and then coming in to a warm kitchen where Ida, in her housedress and apron, waited to pass out hot biscuits and gravy, over eggs. She changed to a wrap-around apron on canning days, when a whole day might be spent snapping beans or peeling tomatoes.

After Dee died, Ida put away her apron and moved into town, where she met her second husband, Jim, at a dance. They enjoyed life together until he died, when they were well into their nineties. Ida, now ninety-five, still enjoys life, though she doesn't cook anymore, even for herself. But she can occasionally be found sweeping the patio of her assisted living residence, sometimes wearing a pretty white apron. The shady yard where Ida made her playhouse is now under the waters of Table Rock Lake, near Branson, Missouri.

Thanks to Claire Henry for assisting with Grandma Ida's interview.

Gotcha Covered: A Legacy of Service and Protection

The Nurses' Apron Partnership

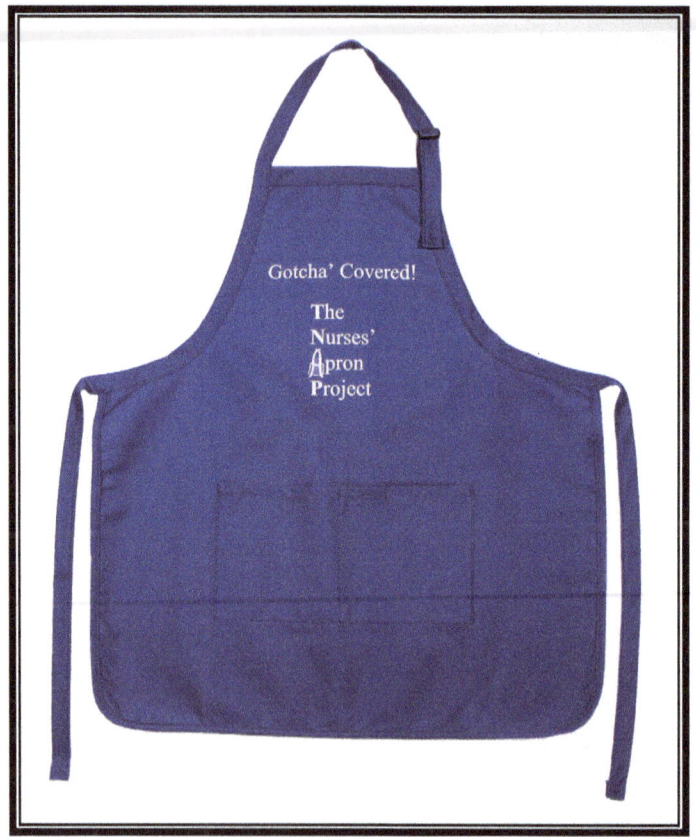

This limited edition blue canvas apron bearing the original logo of TNAP was created in 2008 to raise donations from our authors for the web site.

The Nurses' Apron Partnership

Ginger T. Manley

In the fall of 2006, a group of nurses, who had graduated together from Vanderbilt University forty years earlier, gathered in Nashville for their class reunion. A series of events occurred over the course of that weekend, and in the ensuing weeks that led to the formation of The Nurses' Apron Project, now known as The Nurses' Apron Partnership (TNAP). It is the mission of TNAP to assist nurses in providing health care services, which might not otherwise be available.

This effort initially involved fifty nurses from fifteen states and from Kenya, who joined under the symbolic power of aprons to produce this book and to become a donor portal—a doorway—through which nurses and people who admire the work of nurses can pass, on their way to donating to a microcredit organization in support of nurses in Kenya. TNAP is a grassroots organization, unaffiliated with any group.

TNAP was inspired by the vision of Poppy Buchanan, a nurse in Nashville, who in 1999 began to support Susan Kaburu, a nurse in Kenya who needed basic supplies for her clinic. Within two years of meeting Susan in Nairobi, Poppy had helped supply everything Susan needed. Since then, Poppy has helped Susan found the Samaria Maternity Home in central Kenya, which has become the prototypical nurse-managed health care clinic in that region of the country. In 2003, Poppy, along with several of her nursing friends, colleagues, and family, founded Burning Bush, Inc., a nonprofit, microcredit organization, which has subsequently supported seven entrepreneurial microenterprises in the area. Without Poppy's work, many mothers and children in that region might not be alive today.

Poppy had taught the class of '66, during our public health rotation in Williamson County, TN. When she received the Alumni Award of Excellence at the 2006 Vanderbilt School of Nursing reunion, the members of the class of '66 were thrilled to be there for that honor.

Later that day, several class members, who were attending another reunion event, adopted vintage aprons from a collection passed on to me by my Aunt Katherine Maloney of Telford, TN, who had recently moved from her family farm into a retirement apartment. The vintage aprons inspired stories and other creative legacies in their adopters, and eventually other nurses joined the core group to contribute their submissions, based on an apron adoption. In 2008, the apron submissions and the professionally photographed images of the aprons were collected into an anthology, illuminating the role of the humble apron in the lives of women, and in the lives of nurses. Some of the submissions are inspirational, some humorous, and some evocative of deeply held memories of love and nurturing. All proceeds from the sale of this book are being donated to Burning Bush, Inc. www.burningbushkenya.org

As far as we know, there has not been another grassroots nursing organization with a similar mission, vision, or product. We hope and expect that nurses worldwide, as well as other interested people, will want to be a part of this effort. Nursing has historically been about providing care to those who cannot, at the moment, care for themselves. TNAP continues that tradition forward into the twenty-first century.

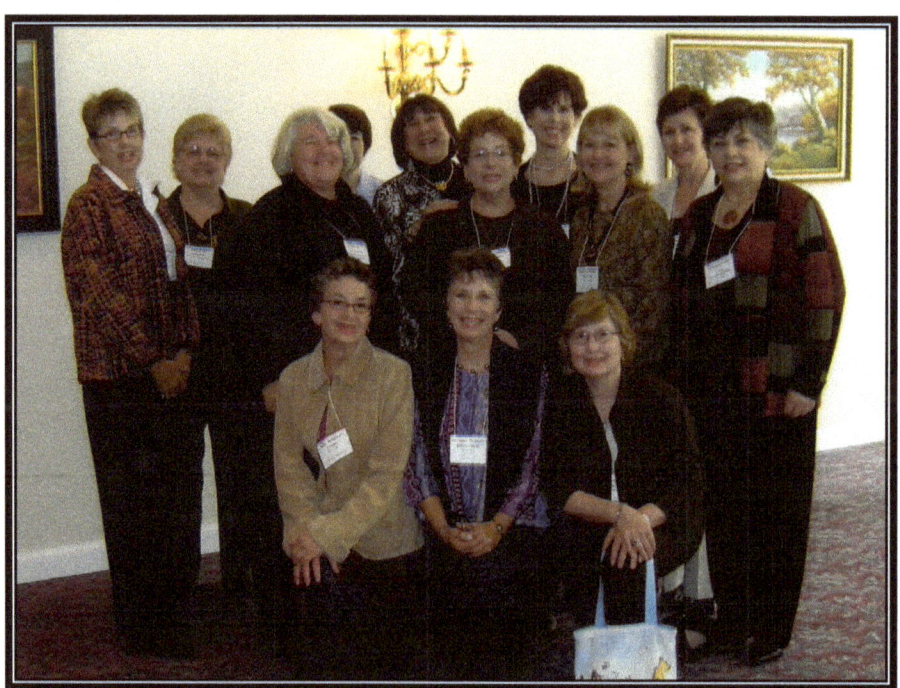

Vanderbilt University School of Nursing Class of 1966 at 40th Class Reunion
Front row: (L–R) Sally Reinhart Crowe, Suzanne Hopkins Blievernicht, Cynthia Fielder Diamond.
Back row: (L–R) Ginger T. Manley, Sally Yeagley, Marilyn Bache Sonnenberg, Cindy Monroe (almost hidden), Sara Jeanne Wells, Ellen E. McGeady, Marti Mueller Daniel, Marilyn Hobbs McAtee, Linda Scott Herzfeld, Donna Cadwallader Miller

Acknowledgments

I did not set out to write a book about aprons, or to start a movement based on aprons. Both of these events found me, and having found me they would not let go. There have been many times when I wished they would move on, away from me, and find someone else to take hostage. Along the way, however, I fell in love with aprons and their stories, and I began to imagine tying together the aprons, the stories, and the experiences of nurses in the United States with those of nurses in Kenya. I am forever grateful to Poppy Buchanan, who taught me as a nursing student in 1965 and 1966. In 2006, after my retirement from nursing, Poppy again came into my life and gifted me with the opportunity to rediscover why I had always loved being a nurse.

I have had three distinct careers as a nurse—first as a hospital-based, intensive care nurse, then as a nurse-practitioner, before hardly anybody knew what that was. My third career, as a psychiatric nurse specialist, took hold in 1981 when I did an internship with Carol Etherington. While my association with Carol since then has been more indirect than direct, Carol always seems to turn up and ask me a question or make a comment that completely turns my life around. In the fall of 2006, after I had been retired for two years, Carol asked me how I was enjoying my retirement and I blurted out that I needed something more than golf and gardening to fill my life. I had not known until then that I harbored such a thought, and Carol quietly said, "I'm sure something will come along." It did. Within a month, The Nurses' Apron Partnership was beginning. Thanks, Carol.

Just as I could not have possibly assembled, much less worn, the first apron I sewed in eighth-grade home economics without the aid, assistance, and encouragement of several people, so I could not have put together this anthology without a great deal of assistance. My classmates from the Vanderbilt University School of Nursing, class of 1966, have always been special to me, and especially so during the conception and delivery of this book. It was they, gathered at my house that night in October 2006, who began telling apron stories, and as I listened, the possibility of finding some way of recording those stories first took root. Especially, I am grateful to my classmates Marti Daniel and Suzanne Blievernicht. Marti has walked (literally) miles with me on this journey—critiquing, querying, supporting, and adding her rich background in the history of feminist politics to my attempts to understand what it was about these aprons that we needed to say. It was Marti who suggested the title for the book, much to my delight. She invited her husband, Rod, to do the photographs, and I was amazed when he said yes. Then as Marti and I helped him to do the shoots, I saw him fall in love with the aprons, too. Many, many thanks to Marti and Rod. Suzanne has always been willing to listen, to critique, to share, to edit, to offer suggestions. She has comforted me when I was discouraged and lifted me up with humor when I was down. Hugs, Suzie2Fish.

In addition to the twenty VUSN classmates who started and the nineteen who ultimately stayed with this process as creative contributors, two other classmates also played a huge part through their financial generosity—Jerry Vaughn Kline and, most especially, Elaine Harrell McConnaughay, donated money to help us get started. Thanks!

Several women in the Middle Tennessee community helped me in an advisory capacity. Many thanks to Daisy King, Bets Ramsey, and Sandra Roberts for your continuing interest and suggestions. Avis Smith in South Australia, whom I have never met, offered the first peek into how aprons could be studied in a scholarly way. When she described to me how she had been inspired to pursue her graduate studies about aprons by her experiences observing nurses in aprons in the Australian bush, I was hooked to learn more. Thanks, Avis, for your generosity of time and spirit as this book was being conceived.

I had never edited a book, nor did I have any idea of how to take this from the idea stage to completion, but I am fortunate to have a cadre of other writers in the Williamson County Council for the Written Word (CWW) in Franklin, TN. Many of these people attend a writers' critique group with me every other week, and they either heard me read, or at my invitation read themselves, many of the pieces that make up this anthology. Thanks to this entire group, and especially to Judith Walter, Len Walker, and Vickie Clasby for helping me see the strengths (or not) and the possibilities of the submissions, when they were in first-draft mode. Your honesty about this project was invaluable. As the work was drawing near publication, I recruited Suzanne Brunson and Currie Alexander Powers from CWW to help me get it all together. They stepped in like the pros they are, and typed, formatted, edited, and advised until we got a coherent document ready for printing. Wow! You guys are the best.

Along the way, I asked several people to do more than I ever should have asked, in the way of helping me to think about where this book might go. Looking back, my only excuse is "ignorance is bliss." Dr. Vereen Bell in the Department of English at Vanderbilt, patiently read every single submission before there had been one bit of internal editing. He taught me in 2007 and 2008 the same lessons he had taught in 1962—dig deeper and see what you can find. He was always kind and engaging, and I am eternally grateful for his support. Michael Ames at the Vanderbilt University Press read every piece and offered many suggestions, and I am most grateful.

In 2007, as I was trying to get all the aprons adopted, one apron was returned to the fold for re-adoption. By coincidence, that same week, Maxine Arnold Dalton attended a gathering in North Carolina where she was seated with Suzanne Blievernicht, whom she had never met. Upon learning about our effort, Maxine immediately adopted the orphaned apron, wrote a lovely piece, and then painted a watercolor, incorporating her apron as one of several on a clothesline. When she sent the watercolor image to me with her written submission, my jaw dropped. I knew I had found our book cover. Thanks, Maxine.

I have been so blessed to have forty-nine nurses who completed this work. Some were eager to write and gave me their pieces quickly. Others struggled to find even a paragraph, agonizing as though it were a thesis or dissertation. When we needed money to complete the typing, formatting, layout, and all the other million pieces that came up near the end, I reluctantly put out a call for donations, knowing that most of us are struggling in this recession. Within twenty-four hours, more than twenty of the writers had responded with offers of money. Every author seemed genuinely thrilled to be a part of this book, and I appreciate all the encouragement and cooperation you have given me. I have still not met some of you, but I feel like you are a part of my family, both the nursing and the kinship families.

I had always heard it said, "If you need something done, ask a busy person to do it." When I asked Virginia Betts to do the foreword with a very tight timeline for completion, I knew I was asking one of the busiest persons on the planet (think Tennessee's budget woes) to take on one more thing. She responded within the day that she would love to do it, and she made it possible for us to meet our deadline with room to spare. I am so grateful, Ginna.

Stacey Irvin has been a charm as our graphic artist and web designer, never once complaining about all my ignorance about what she does. She took the initial logo, which Marti, Suzanne, and I had drawn out, and she brought it to life. We are so glad to have you on our team, Stacey. Dianne Green stepped in at just the right moment to help me see how we could bring this book to the public. She revamped our web site and proofread every word of this manuscript! Thanks!

Finding Published by Westview, Inc. almost in my own back yard was truly a fortunate experience. In my first meeting with her, I asked Mary Catherine Nelson at Westview to hold my hand all the way through this, and she did so with grace and humor, occasionally reminding me to "Breathe, Ginger." It has been a joyful experience and I am still breathing. Thanks for believing in this wonderful book from day one, M.C.

My husband, John Manley, has been my most important supporter as I have put this all together. John will probably never truly understand my obsession with aprons, or with words for that matter, but he has loved me through all of this, and he is my biggest ally. Thanks, J.G. Forty-two years, and still going strong!

Ultimately, I am grateful to all the nurses who have come before me and to those who have followed. Good nursing care really does matter, whether in Tennessee or in Kenya.

Ginger T. Manley
Franklin, TN
June 4, 2009

References and Bibliography

"19th Century Girls' Aprons." [online] Available at: http://www.flickr.com/groups/vintageaprons/discuss/72157603875138534 (Accessed March 3, 2008)

"#56 Mary Morris Husband." Daughters of Union Veterans of the Civil War 1861–1865 National Web Site. [online] Available at: http://www.duvcw.org/pa/history58.html (Accessed March 3, 2008)

"A10336 Man's work apron." Powerhouse Museum Collection. [online] Available at: http://www.powerhousemuseum.com/collection/database/?irn=169574 (Accessed March 3, 2008)

Apron Strings lyrics. [online] Available at: http://www.hotlyrics.net/lyrics/E/Elvis_Presley/Apron_Strings.html (Accessed March 4, 2008)

"Apron strings: ties to the past." Michigan Historical Museum. [online] Available at: http://www.hal.state.mi.us/mhc/museum/explore/museums/hismus/special/aprons/samples.html (Accessed June 2, 2009)

"Apron strings: ties to the past." Mid-America Arts Alliance and Exhibits USA. [online] Available at: http://www.maaa.org/exhi_usa/exhibitions/archive/apron/apron.html (Accessed March 3, 2008)

"Aprons in the Middle Ages and Renaissance." [online] Available at: http://www.larsdatter.com/aprons.htm (Accessed May 28, 2009)

"Army medics train at Miami Trauma Center." [online] Available at: http://www.wjla.com/news/stories/1007/467022.html (Accessed March 3, 2008)

Barr, J. M. B., Schiska, A. "Radiologic safety: historical perspectives and contemporary recommendations." *Journal of Radiology Nursing*. [online] Available at: http://linkinghub.elsevier.com/retrieve/pii/S1546084305000064 (Accessed March 3, 2008)

Bartle, R. "Taranaki stories: the story of Truby King and the Plunkett nurses." [online] Available at: http://www.pukeariki.com/en/stories/scienceAndMedicine/plunketnurse.htm (Accessed March 3, 2008)

Blievernicht, S. [e-mail to Ginger T. Manley] December 2, 2006. Available at e-mail: info@thenursesapronpartnership.com

Bostridge, M. *Florence Nightingale: The Making of an Icon.* New York: Farrar, Strous, and Giroux; 2008.

Brontë, A. *The Tenant of Wildfell Hall.* 1848. Oxford World Classics, Herbert Rosengarten, ed. New York: Oxford University Press; 1992

Ceci, S. J., Williams, W., Barnett, S. M. "Women's underrepresentation in science: sociocultural and biological considerations." *Psychological Bulletin.* [online] Available at: http://www.apa.org/journals/releases/bul1352218.pdf (Accessed June 1, 2009)

Cheney, J. *Aprons: Icons of the American Home.* Philadelphia: Running Press Book Publishers; 2000.

Chevalier, T. *Girl with the Pearl Earring.* New York: Plume; 1999.

Clegg, R. I. "Was William Shaekspeare a Freemason?" [online] Available at: http://www.masonicdictionary.com/shakespeare.html (Accessed May 28, 2009)

Colgrove, D. "Free pattern and directions for sewing a dish liquid bottle apron." [online] Available at: http://sewing.about.com/od/aprons/ss/soapapron.htm (Accessed March 3, 2008)

"Collecting and recollecting: gifts from the recent past." University of Iowa Health Care. [online] Available at: http://www.uihealthcare.com/depts/medmuseum/galleryexhibits/collectingfrompast/nursing/nursing.html (Accessed March 4, 2008)

Craik, J. "Cultural studies and history: a story of flirtation and poaching." [online] Available at: http://www.nla.gov.au/events/history/papers/Jennifer_Craik.html (Accessed March 3, 2008)

DePree, T. *Aprons on a Clothesline.* Colorado Springs, CO WaterBrook Press; 2005.

DiMaggio, E. M. "Some suggestions for the female re-enactor." [online] Available at: http://www.missselliesemporium.com/articles/why.shtml (Accessed March 3, 2008)

Donahue, M. P. *Nursing: The Finest Art: An Illustrated History.* St. Louis: The C.V. Mosby Company; 1985.

Driver, S.W. "A cherished apron." [online] Available at: http://www.stretcher.com/stories/04/04jun28g.cfm (Accessed March 3, 2008)

Ferns, T., Chojnacka, I. "Angels and swingers, matrons and sinners: nursing stereotypes." *British Journal of Nursing* [online] Available at: http://www.internurse.com/cgi-bin/go.pl/library/abstract.html?uid=19947 (Accessed March 4, 2008)

"Vintage aprons." Flickr group. [online] Available at: http://www.flickr.com/groups/vintageaprons/ (Accessed March 3, 2008)

Ford, L. "A look back: Worcester Hahnemann Hospital School of Nursing." [online] Available at: http://pictureyoshi.tripod.com/our_history.htm (Accessed March 3, 2008)

Freeland, S. "Nursing uniforms throughout history." [online] Available at: http://ezinearticles.com/?Nursing-Uniforms-Through-History&id=403057 (Accessed March 3, 2008)

Geisel, E. *The Apron Book: Making, Wearing, and Sharing a Bit of Cloth and Comfort.* Kansas City: Andrews McMeel Publishing; 2006.

Gibson, L. R. "Beyond the apron: archetypes, stereotypes, and alternative portrayals of mothers in children's literature." *Children's Literature Association Quarterly.* 13:4, 177–181.

Goldman, M. "The string that tie, a short tale of aprons." [online] Available at: http://www.betterbaking.com/viewArticle.php?article_id=84 (Accessed March 8, 2008)

Grandma's Apron. [online] Available at: http://www.womensfunnyvideos.com/Inspirational/grandma-apron.htm (Accessed June 1, 2009)

Green R. "Nurse dolls show how the profession has evolved." [online] Available at: http://allnurses.com/nursing-news/nurse-dolls-show-66926.html (Accessed March 3, 2008)

Greenhill, E. D., Browning, L. *A 100 Year History of the Tennessee Nurses' Association: 1905–2005.* Nashville: Tennessee Nurses' Foundation, 2006.

Harwood, P. "Tippetts to scrubs—a brief history of UK nursing uniforms." [online] Available at: http://dyk.homestead.com/Philswords.html (Accessed March 3, 2008)

"Haute Hostess Aprons by Elizabeth Scokin." [online] Available at: http://www.hautehostessaprons.com/products/calendar/index.asp (Accessed June 11, 2009)

Heather, I. Book review: *Daring to Care: American Nursing and Second Wave Feminism.* [online] Available at: http://feministreview.blogspot.com/search/label/nursing (Accessed March 3, 2008)

"History of Marquette General Hospital." St. Luke's Hospital Training School for Nurses. [online] Available at: http://www.mgh.org/history/nursesch.htm (Accessed March 3, 2008)

Hoffer, V. "The Mormon temple endowment homepage." [online] Available at: http://www.lds-mormon.com/veilworker/endowment1.shtml (Accessed March 3, 2008)

"Hospital uniforms." Canadian Nursing History Collection. [online] Available at: http://www.civilization.ca/cmc/exhibitions/tresors/nursing/nccat01e.shtml (Accessed March 3, 2008)

Hymowitz, K. S. "Red-state feminism." *City Journal* [online] Available at: http://www.city-journal.org/2008/eon0908kh.html (Accessed February 12, 2009)

Image of child dressed in Florence Nightingale costume. [online] Available at: http://www.platinumcostumes.com/index.php?main_page=popup_image&pID=1612 (Accessed March 3, 2008)

Image of George Washington's Masonic apron. [online] Available at: http://www.utlm.org/images/masonictemplearticle/thecraftanditssymbols_p11.gif (Accessed March 3, 2008)

Jaret, P. *Nurse: A World of Care.* Atlanta: Emory University Press; 2008.

Judi. "The history of aprons." [online] Available at: http://www.stitchesinfaith.com/historyofaprons.htm (Accessed March 3, 2008)

Karol, A. "The no $$ apron gallery is up." [online] Available at: http://angrychicken.typepad.com/tieoneon/ (Accessed March 3, 2008 and May 17, 2009)

Kay, H. *Apron On, Apron Off.* New York: Scholastic Book Services; 1968.

Kirchheimer, S. (2009). "50 thrifty ideas." *AARPTheMagazine*, Washington, D.C. May–June 2009: 24, 26, 31.

Klinefelter, E. "Twenty-five years." [online] Available at: http://beckerexhibits.wustl.edu/mowihsp/words/KlinefelterSpeech.htm (Accessed March 3, 2008)

Kneeland, N. *Aprons and House Dresses.* [online] Available at: http://hearth.library.cornell.edu/cgi/t/text/text-idx?c=hearth;idno=4400047 (Accessed May 13, 2009)

"Lizzie Andrew Borden Quotes." [online] Available at: http://www.brainyquote.com/quotes/authors/l/lizzie_andrew_borden.html (Accessed March 4, 2008)

Lucy. "The sassy apron swap." [online] Available at: http://sassyapronswap.blogspot.com/2008/01/apron-swap-spring-2008.html (Accessed March 3, 2008)

McCants, K. "Modern June." [online] Available at: http://modernjune.blogspot.com/ (Accessed March 3, 2008 and May 17, 2009)

Maggie. "Apron evangelism." [online] Available at: http://www.hillbillyhousewife.com/apronevangelism.htm (Accessed March 3, 2008)

Malka, S. G. *Daring to Care: American Nursing and Second-Wave Feminism.* Champaign, IL: University of Illinois Press; 2007.

McCall 1169 c. 1944 Vintage apron pattern [online] Available at: http://patternaholic.blogspot.com/2007/11/mccall-1169-c-1944-vinrage-apron.html (Accessed June 3, 2009)

McComb, J. (1971) *The Priceless Gift.* [online] Available at: http://www.elvis.com/elvisology/writings/elvis_pricelessgift.asp (Accessed August 16, 2007)

"Men in aprons." [online] Available at: http://www.meninaprons.net/archives.html (Accessed March 3, 2008)

Mia. "The apron strings." [online] Available at: http://ecomama.blogspot.com/2008/09/apron-strings.html (Accessed May 17, 2009)

"Minidoka hospital workers." Washington State Historical Society digital images. [online] 1994. Available at: http://digitum.washingtonhistory.org/cdm4/browse.php?CISOROOT=/womens&CISOSTART=1,41 (Accessed March 3, 2008)

Modern Butterick apron pattern B6567. [online] Available at: http://www.butterick.com/web/shop.cgi?s.item.B6567 (Accessed June 3, 2009)

Modern McCall's apron pattern [online] Available at: http://www.mccallpattern.com/item/M3979.htm (Accessed June 3, 2009)

Mount, T. "Medieval housewives." [online] Available at: http://www.richardiii.net/medieval%20life.htm (Accessed March 3, 2008)

My Byrd House. [online] Available at: http://mybyrdhouse.blogspot.com/ (Accessed March 3, 2008 and May 17, 2009)

Neels, B. (1970). *Nurse in Holland* (original title: *Amazon in an Apron*) Amazon.com [online] Available at: http://www.amazon.com/Nurse-Holland-Original-Title-Harlequin/dp/B0012GCXGU/ref (Accessed February 22, 2009)

North Carolina Baptist Hospital School of Nursing Archives [online] Available at: http://ewake.wfubmc.edu:88/library/archives/exhibits/nursing/uniforms.htm (Accessed March 3, 2008)

"Nurse Uniforms." [online] Available at: http://www.nursingdaily.co.uk/nurse-uniforms.php (Accessed March 3, 2008)

"Nurses and the U.S. Navy, 1917–1919—Red Cross and Army nurses' uniforms." Department of the Navy—Naval Historical Center. [online] Available at: http://www.history.navy.mil/photos/prs-tpic/nurses/nrs-e8d.htm (Accessed March 3, 2008)

"Nurses Graduating from St. Mark's Hospital." Westminster College Archives. [online] Available at: http://content.lib.utah.edu/cdm4/item_viewer.php?CISOROOT=/WC_PhotoCol&CISOPTR=109&CISOBOX=1&REC=6 (Accessed March 3, 2008)

"Nurses Uniforms History" [online] Available at: http://nurse.lifetips.com/cat/59404/nursing-history/ (Accessed March 3, 2008)

Oliver, L. (1974). "Women in aprons: the female stereotype in children's readers." *The Elementary School Journal*, 74: 5, 253–259.

Patterns Vintage Aprons. [online] Available at: http://www.sovintagepatterns.com/page/page/1663215.htm (Accessed June 3, 2009)

Pearson, G. S. *Aprons on a Clothesline*: book review. *Perspectives in Psychiatric Care*. [online] Available at: http://www3.interscience.wiley.com/journal/118727920/abstract? (Accessed May 26, 2009)

Peay, P. "Feminism's fourth wave." *Utne Reader.* [online] Available at: http://www.utne.com/2005-03-01/feminisms-fourth-wave.aspx (Accessed March 3, 2008)

"Radiation safety in the endoscopy setting." Society of Gastroenterology Nurses and Associates. [online] Available at: http://www.sgna.org/Resources/guidelines/guideline2.cfm (Accessed March 3, 2008)

"Sexy apron day." [online] Available at: http://www.etsy.com/shop.php?user_id=5292030 (Accessed March 3, 2008, May 17, 2009)

Shawnee. "Flirty apron swap." [online] Available at: http://flirtyapronswap.blogspot.com/ (Accessed March 3, 2008 and May 17, 2009)

Shortridge, R. D. "The meaning of the apron." [online] Available at: http://www.absalom.com/mormon/contrib/shortridge/apron.html (Accessed March 3, 2008)

Smith, A. (2002) "Making a statement with an apron." [online] Available at: http://www.cccs.uq.edu.au/events/fashion/abstracts/smith.php (Accessed March 3, 2008)

Smith, A. *The Language of Aprons: Signifiers of Femininity.* University of South Adelaide: Unpublished Master's thesis; 2003.

Smith, A. [e-mail to Ginger T. Manley] March 6, 2008. Available at e-mail: info@thenursesapronpartnership.com

South Carolina Department of Mental Health. "Comparing the mental health of the past to the mental health in the present." [online] Available at: http://www.state.sc.us/dmh/then_now.htm (Accessed March 3, 2008)

SPmag admin. "Apron strings keep women out of math fields." *Smart People* [online] Available at: http://www.smartpeoplemagazine.com/2009/04/apron-strings-keep-women-out-of-math-fields/ (Accessed May 30, 2009)

Stein, A. P. "Northern volunteer nurses of America's Civil War." [online] Available at: http://www.historynet.com/culture/womens_history/3025866.html?page=3&c=y (Accessed January 17, 2007)

Tammy. "Apron links." [online] Available at: http://lovetocrochetandknit.blogspot.com/2006/05/apron-links.html (Accessed March 3, 2008)

Thayer, C. [e-mail to Ginger T. Manley]. May 27, 2009. Available at e-mail: info@thenursesapronpartnership.com

"The apron festival concludes." National Radio Life Matters. [online] Available at: http://www.abc.net.au/rn/lifematters/index/subjects_People_2005.htm (Accessed March 3, 2008)

The Holy Bible. Revised Standard Version. New York: Thomas Nelson & Sons. 1952.

Thompson, J. "A working woman's dress revisited." [online] Available at: http://www.festiveattyre.com/research/working.html (Accessed March 3, 2008)

Trivett, T. *Grandma's Apron*. [online] Available at: http://tinatrivett.blogspot.com/2007/08/grandmas-apron.html (Accessed June 1, 2009)

Trottman, M. "Once dowdy, the apron ascends to costly kitchen couture." *Wall Street Journal* [online] Available at: http://www.apronmemories.com/pdf/wsj081205.pdf (Accessed February 12, 2009)

US Patent 5318507. Detachable back, belt, apron method. [online] Available at: http://www.patentstorm.us/patents/5318507/description.html (Accessed March 3, 2008)

"What's the big deal about 'naughty nurse' images in the media?" The Center for Nursing Advocacy [online] Available at: http://www.nursingadvocacy.org/faq/naughty_nurse.html (Accessed March 3, 2008)

"Why do QA Army nurses wear grey dresses and berets?" [online] Available at: http://www.qaranc.co.uk/qarancgreyuniform.php (Accessed March 3, 2008)

Wiggins, P. "Collectors tie one on with vintage aprons: aprons from Victorian to Mid-Century." [online] Available at: http://antiques.about.com/od/textilesandquilts/a/aa112502.htm (Accessed March 3, 2008)

Worts, F. R. "The apron and its symbolism." [online] Available at: http://freemasonry.bcy.ca/aqc/apron.html (Accessed March 3, 2008)

Yarbrough, A. "A history of 1950s aprons." [online] Available at: http://www.associatedcontent.com/article/391415/a_history_of_1950s_aprons.html?cat=37 (Accessed March 3, 2008)

Zwerdling, M. *Postcards of Nursing: A Worldwide Tribute*. Philadelphia: Lippincott Williams & Wilkins; 2004.

Zwerdling, M., [e-mail to Ginger T. Manley] April 12, 2008. Available at e-mail: info@thenursesapronpartnership.com

TWENTY-THREE *Gotcha Covered* CONTRIBUTORS

gathered at Miss Daisy's Kitchen in Franklin, TN, on Oct. 24, 2009 for the debut party for the book.

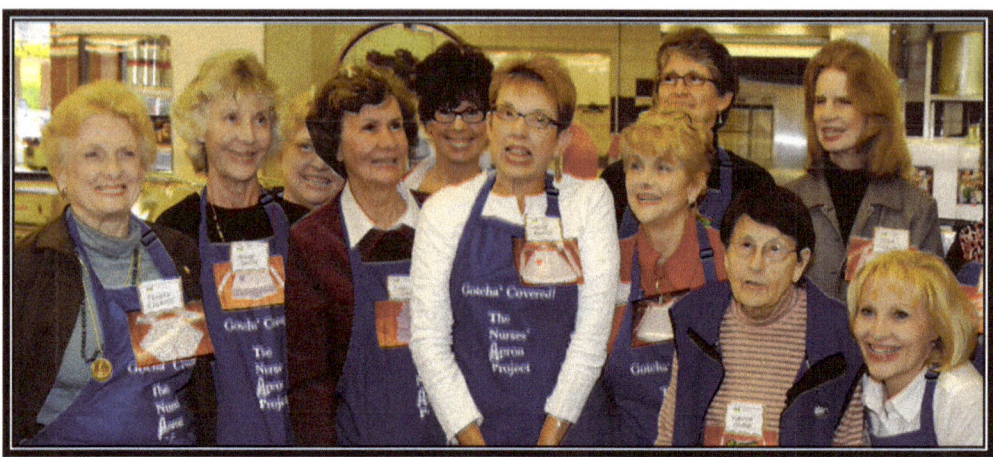

Frances Edwards, Maxine Dalton, Sally Yeagley, Carol Dixon, Marti Daniel, Ginger Manley, Karen Starr, Bev Byram, Virginia George, Lydia Grubb, Amanda Pendley

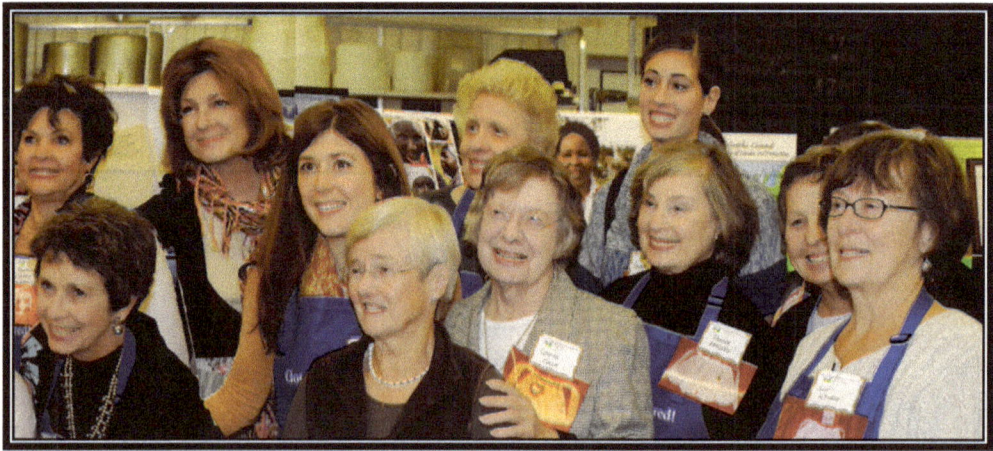

Barbara Vinson, Suzanne Blievernicht, Carol Etherington, Krista Koleas, Eileen Richardson, Poppy Buchanan, Louise Colln, Brooke Faught, Donna Maddox, Marceleen Alford, Sue Wilson, not pictured, Mary Gresham Barr

Photo by Rod Daniel

CONTRIBUTING AUTHORS

Sharon Adkins lives in Graball, TN. She has a BSN (1970) from the University of Minnesota and an MSN (1988) from Vanderbilt University. She has spent her career in a variety of roles, from neonatal intensive care to director of the Center for Parish Nursing & Health Ministries. She currently serves as the Executive Director of the Tennessee Nurses' Association.

Marceleen Rodes Alford lives in Nashville, TN. She has a BSN from Vanderbilt University (1962). She has practiced most of her professional life in Emergency Rooms and Recovery Rooms.

Mary Gresham Buchanan Barr lives in Nashville, TN. She graduated from Texas Christian University with a BSN (1987). Her nursing career has included hospice and summer camp nursing. Currently she is getting a Masters in Nursing at Belmont University. In her spare time, she enjoys being at home with three teenagers, ages seventeen, fifteen, and thirteen, a husband, and five cats and dogs.

Patricia Vuleta Spence Benn lives in Hannibal, MO. She graduated from Allegheny General Hospital School of Nursing in 1967. She has practiced as a medical and surgical nurse in hospitals and in industry. She is now retired.

Suzanne Hopkins Blievernicht lives in Asheville, NC. She has a BSN from Vanderbilt University (1966) and an MN from Emory University (1969). Her forty-three-year nursing practice includes being a Clinical Specialist, and working in critical care, as a nurse educator, in hospice, and as a Healing Touch Practitioner. She has also worked as a therapy dog trainer. She is a mother, medical practice coordinator, has published short stories and poems, and has a memoir in progress. She loves living on a small farm with her husband, fly-fishing, golf, camping, and being a nurse.

Poppy Pickering Buchanan lives in Nashville, TN. She has a BSN (1961) from Vanderbilt University. She has practiced and taught public health nursing, and has managed a real estate portfolio. Since 1999, she has been involved with Burning Bush Inc, a non-profit organization chartered to support the work of a Kenyan Nurse/midwife, and to invest in that community through programs, including micro-lending groups.

Sharron Stewart Burch lives in Brandon, MS. She graduated from Vanderbilt University in 1966 with a BSN, and the University of Mississippi Medical Center in 1975 with an MN. She has practiced most of her professional life as a nursing instructor in the ADN programs at two different Community Colleges in MS. She retired from the Division of Medicaid in March 2005.

Beverly Byram lives in Nashville, TN. She graduated from the University of Tennessee (AAN) in 1975 and Vanderbilt University (MSN) in 1992. Her career encompasses adult medical/surgical and pediatric psychiatric nursing. Since becoming a nurse-practitioner, her passion has been working with HIV patients, especially women. She founded the OB/HIV clinic at Vanderbilt, where she serves as Director of Women's Health.

Judith B. Collins lives in Richmond, VA. She graduated from the University of North Carolina with a BSN (1962) and from Boston University with an MS (1968). She completed the Women's Health Nurse-Practitioner Program at Medical College of Virginia/ Virginia Commonwealth University (1975). Her career in nursing has focused on women's health and health policy as a nurse-practitioner, faculty member, and administrator of a comprehensive Women's Clinic. Two special experiences were service on the Hospital Ship HOPE, and as a Robert Wood Johnson Health Policy Fellow in Congress. Since retirement in 2000, she volunteers on several community boards, and enjoys grandchildren and travel.

Louise Colln lives in Franklin, TN. She graduated from the Nashville General Hospital School of Nursing in 1945. Her nursing experience varied from bedside to executive. She has five novels published, and is completing another one. She has poetry and short stories in magazines, online, and in print anthologies.

Sally Reinhart Crowe lives in North Liberty, IA. She graduated from Vanderbilt University with a BSN in 1966. She is presently retired from nursing and actively participating in prairie restoration on her rural home.

Maxine Arnold Dalton lives in Spring Creek, NC. She received her BSN (1962) from Vanderbilt University and her PhD (1985) in Industrial Organizational Psychology from the University of South Florida. She is retired and enjoys hiking, quilting, painting, and gardening. She volunteers extensively and chairs the Governor's Council on Parks, Parkways, and National Forests.

Marti Mueller Daniel lives in Franklin, TN. She has a BSN (1966) from Vanderbilt University and an MA (1996) in Counseling Psychology with an emphasis in Depth Psychology from Pacifica Graduate Institute, Carpinteria, CA. As a nurse, she specialized in medical and geriatric nursing. In her capacity as a counselor, she was a California MFCC intern, studied Integrative Body

Psychotherapy (IBP), and utilized sand tray, movement, and art therapies in her practice. Presently she lives in the country where she is pursuing oil painting, writing, and documenting her family genealogy.

Libby Dayani lives in Brentwood, TN. She earned her BSN (1971) and MSN (1972) from Vanderbilt. She worked first as a family nurse-practitioner, then as a nurse entrepreneur and senior healthcare executive. Now retired, she enjoys reading, gardening, and playing as often as possible with her three grandsons.

Cynthia Fielder Diamond lives in Shawnee, KS. She graduated from Vanderbilt University (BSN) in 1966 and practiced as a nurse for forty years in Tennessee and Kansas. An Oncology Certified Nurse (OCN), she worked for twenty-eight years on the Hematology-Oncology unit at the University of Kansas Hospital. She retired in 2006.

Carol E. Dixon lives in Hot Springs, NC. She has a BSN from Wright State University in Ohio (1976), and an MSN from Ohio State (1978). In 1978, she and a colleague started Hospice of Dayton, Ohio. Since retirement in 1996, several of her short stories and essays have been published.

Frances McGaughy Edwards lives in Nashville, TN. She graduated from Vanderbilt University with a BSN (1953) and an MSN (1975). She has practiced nursing in many settings, including sexual health education, vascular surgery and energetic healing. At present, she holds an adjunct faculty position at Vanderbilt, and is involved with Healing Touch research for breast cancer patients.

Carol Etherington lives in Nashville, TN. She graduated with a BSN from Catherine Spaulding College, now Spaulding University, and received her MSN from Vanderbilt University in 1975, specializing in psychiatric nursing. She has spent her career focusing on the mental health needs of trauma survivors, working and teaching worldwide. She is the past president of Doctors without Borders, and was the 2007 recipient of the Outstanding Alumnus Award from Vanderbilt Alumni Association.

Diane Carlson Evans lives in Helena, MT. She graduated from St. Barnabas Hospital School of Nursing in 1967. The six years she spent in the Army Nurse Corps during the Vietnam War shaped her life-long career in advocacy work for veterans. She is a peace activist, author, educator, consultant, and passionate about nursing's legacy of healing and hope.

Brooke Faught lives in Brentwood, Tennessee. She is a 2001 graduate of the Ohio State University College of Nursing, and a 2003 graduate of the University of Pennsylvania School Of Nursing where she completed her graduate training. She founded the Women's Institute for Sexual Health (WISH) in Nashville in 2005 and now serves as its clinical director.

Jennie Maddra Fleshood lives in Vero Beach, FL. She graduated from Stuart Circle Hospital School of Nursing in 1963. Her nursing career was focused in gastroenterology. She is now retired.

Lisa Fournace lives in Mt. Juliet, TN. She graduated with a BS from Middle Tennessee State University in 1995, and has an MSN from Vanderbilt University (2004). She practices as a women's health nurse-practitioner, specializing in urogynecology and pelvic pain.

Margaret Kuehnle Fulton lives in Ferriday, LA. She graduated from Vanderbilt University with a BSN in 1966. Her early nursing experience was in coronary and medical intensive care, and she was a public health nurse for eight years. She has been a Health Ministry Consultant and Parish Nurse Coordinator for the Mississippi Conference of the United Methodist Church, and is still a Parish Nurse.

Virginia M. George lives in Nashville, TN. She has a BSN (1947) and an MS in Psychology (1972, Peabody) from Vanderbilt University, and an MSN (1973) from the University of Alabama-Birmingham. She was a faculty member at Northeast Louisiana State College (1963–1964) and at Vanderbilt University School of Nursing from 1956–1958, and again from 1964–1990, serving as director of the graduate Family Nurse-Practitioner program at Vanderbilt until her retirement.

Lydia Luttrell Grubb lives in Nashville, TN. She graduated from the University of Tennessee with a BSN (1968) and from Vanderbilt University with an MSN (1973). She has taught fundamentals of nursing in several college settings, and works as a supervisor in the Centennial Women's Hospital in Nashville.

Linda Scott Herzfeld lives in Montgomery, AL. She has a BSN (1966) from Vanderbilt University. During her career, she served as a public health nurse, infant care business owner, and nurse manager and compliance specialist with the American Red Cross. She is now retired.

Susan Kaburu lives in Nyeri, Kenya. She graduated in 1977 from Kenyatta National Hospital School of Nursing. She is the matron and owner of the Samaria Maternity Center in Nyeri. Her main interests away from work are family, church, and friends. She loves to sing.

Krista Koleas lives in Nashville, TN. She has a BS degree from Belmont University (1999) and an MSN (2003) from Vanderbilt University. She currently practices at Nashville Skin and Cancer dermatology clinic. She also enjoys giving her time and nursing skills as a volunteer to Siloam Family Health Center, and various overseas mission opportunities.

Kathleen S. Lewis lives in Marietta, GA. She has a BSN from Vanderbilt University (1966), an MS in counseling from Georgia State University, and has taken the core content as a Marriage and Family Therapist from the University of Georgia. She is a Licensed Professional Counselor, Certified Medical Psychotherapist, and Stephen Minister. She runs a counseling ministry, Celebrate Life. She is widely published in professional and lay journals, and is the author of *Celebrate Life . . . New Attitudes for Living with Chronic Illness*, in its 3rd printing, and *Prayer Without Ceasing . . . Breath Prayers*. She speaks around the country to patient and professional groups on successful living with chronic illness.

Linda Schlesinger Mabry lives in Tallahassee, FL. She has a BSN (1966) from Vanderbilt University. She practiced clinical nursing at the Veterans Administration Hospital in Nashville, TN, and briefly in New Haven, CT, followed by a break from the workforce for twelve busy years, rearing her daughters. In a second career of twenty years (job-sharing), she developed and presented training for the State of Florida to assisted living facilities and adult family-care home administrators, in a fourteen county area. She is now retired.

Donna Maddox lives on Longboat Key, FL. She is a graduate of Radford University, and has a BSN from Vanderbilt University (1961). She is president of Marketing & Business Consultants and is a life member of International Association of Business Communicators. She is the author of the book *Message of the Cameos*.

Ginger T. Manley lives in Franklin, TN. She has a BSN (1966) and an MSN from Vanderbilt University (1981), in psychiatric nursing. She has practiced as an advanced practice nurse, specializing in sex therapy for most of her career, and presently is an Associate in the Department of Psychiatry, Vanderbilt University Medical School, and a Clinical Professor of Nursing at Vanderbilt University School of Nursing. Her passions are gardening, writing, and golf.

Marilyn Hobbs McAtee lives in Nashville, IN. She graduated in 1966 from Vanderbilt University with a BSN. She has practiced most of her career as a Community Health Nurse, and is currently the Director of the Brown Co. Health Support Clinic, a clinic for the uninsured and underserved residents of the county.

Ellen E. McGeady lives in North Charleston, SC. She has a BSN from Vanderbilt University (1966) and an MA in Nursing from Columbia University (1968). She practiced as a clinical specialist in psychiatric nursing in New York City and Chicago, and later worked administratively in the areas of quality management, utilization review, and clinical case management. A long time resident of Illinois, she is currently retired from nursing and designs jewelry.

Judy Tincher Monaco lives in Ormond Beach, FL. She and her husband have a second home in the Paradise Valley, MT. She graduated from Vanderbilt University with a BSN (1966). She has taught nursing-skills courses and administered nursing curriculum at the local community college. After raising her family, she returned to nursing, specializing in pediatrics. She has been involved in many community charities, and received the Jefferson Award for central Florida.

Rebekah Nesbitt lives in Nashville, TN. She graduated from Medical University of South Carolina with a BSN (2004). She also has a degree in Psychology from Vanderbilt University (2002). She has practiced as an RN in the Pediatric Critical Care Unit at Vanderbilt Children's Hospital since finishing nursing school in 2004.

Charlotte Richardson Norwood lives in McLean, VA. She has a BSN (1966) from Vanderbilt University. She is a member of two professional bands, both jazz and Dixieland, which tour nationally and internationally.

Amanda Taylor Pendley lives in Madisonville, KY. She has an MSN from Vanderbilt University (1999). She practices as a psychiatric nurse-practitioner at Trover Health Systems Center for Behavioral Health in Madisonville, Kentucky, and is a clinical instructor at Vanderbilt University School of Nursing.

Mary Jo Reimer lives in northern Kentucky. She graduated from Los Angeles Community College with an ADN (1995). She practiced most of her career in Los Angeles as an AIDS hospice nurse. Currently, she is working part-time as an evening supervisor at St. Charles Care Center.

Marilyn Bache Sonnenberg lives in Mandeville, LA. She holds a BSN (1966) from Vanderbilt University, an MS (1969) from Boston University, and a PhD (1984) from The University of Texas at Dallas. In recognition of her life-long commitment to volunteerism, she received the Outstanding Faculty Service Award from the University of South Carolina in 2000. Now retired, she spent most of her professional career in nursing administration.

Karen L. Starr lives in Nashville, TN. She received a BA from William Woods College (1976), a BSN from the University of Missouri-Columbia (1976), and an MSN from Vanderbilt University

(1983). She has practiced most of her professional life as a psychiatric nurse-practitioner, specializing in addiction and solid organ transplant psychiatry. She teaches at Vanderbilt School of Nursing, and is a faculty member in the School of Medicine, Department of Psychiatry.

Joan Crosland Chapman Sughrue lives in Woodstock, GA. She has a BSN (1969) from the University of South Carolina and an M.Ed. in Clinical Counseling (1982) from The Citadel in Charleston, SC. She has practiced most of her professional life in women's health, and as a certified sex therapist with her late husband, John Sughrue, Jr., M.D. She currently teaches sexuality training workshops for medical, nursing, and mental health professionals.

Barbara Siddens Vinson lives in Bowling Green, KY. She graduated from Vanderbilt University with a BSN in 1966. She has worked predominately in intensive care areas (SICU, CCU, ER, and Cardiac Cath Lab) throughout her nursing career. She currently works as a pre- and post-operative nurse, and plans to retire in 2009.

Sara Jeanne Wells lives in Atlanta, GA. She has a BSN (1966) from Vanderbilt University and an MN (1970) from Emory University. She has worked as a Cardiovascular Clinical Specialist, and in several administrative positions in the North East and South. She has held numerous faculty appointments at colleges and universities throughout the East Coast, and has published four books and numerous articles. Presently, she is a consultant for a small California company.

Myra Wilson Willey lives in Lebanon, TN. She graduated from Vanderbilt University with a BSN in 1966 and an MSSW in 1983 from University of Tennessee. She retired from the V.A. Medical Center in Murfreesboro in 2003. She was employed there for thirty-three years as a nurse and as a medical social worker.

Sue Wilson lives in Franklin, TN. She graduated from Mercy Hospital School of Nursing (1962), University of Michigan Pediatric Nurse-Practitioner Certificate Program (1980), and Sienna Heights College (BAS, 1987). A certified Pediatric Nurse-Practitioner, she spent most of her career in pediatrics. She retired in 1998 as administrator for a large, Michigan, hospital-based, adult and pediatric home health and hospice program. Her published works include "You and the Dying Child" in the collaborative, hospice volunteer source book, *Your Gift*.

Kathleen L. Wolff lives in Nashville, TN. She graduated from the University of South Florida with a degree in Humanities Education in 1975, has an ADN from Tennessee State University (1979), and an MSN from Vanderbilt University (1983). She is a harpist, kayaker, and avid gardener, and has co-written a book about people living with diabetes. She has practiced as a Diabetes Nurse-Practitioner since 1983, and currently works at Vanderbilt University Medical Center.

Dianne Horton Wood lives in Franklin, TN. She graduated from the University of Tennessee with a BSN (1969).

Sally Yeagley lives in Nashville, TN. She graduated from Vanderbilt University with a BSN (1966) and an MSN (1986). She currently enjoys working as a Women's Health Nurse-Practitioner. Other interests include antique shopping, reading, and loving three grandchildren.

Dorothy Vaughan and **Lynne Roggen** were original adopters who were not able to continue to the completion of this book.

Photographic and Illustration Credits

All professional apron photography was done by Rod Daniel

Rod Daniel lives in Franklin, TN. He has a BA from Vanderbilt University (1965). He has produced and directed numerous television shows and motion picture films, including *WKRP in Cincinnati*, *Teen Wolf*, *Like Father Like Son*, *K-9*, *The Super*, and *Beethoven's 2nd*. Since retiring from active filmmaking, he is pursuing a new career as a photographer.

Archival images of nurses are © Zwerdling Nursing Archives. http://www.nursepostcard.com

The original watercolor of aprons on a clothesline was done by **Maxine Arnold Dalton** and submitted by her along with her essay for this book.

TNAP graphic design was done by Stacey Irvin

Stacey Irvin lives in Nashville, TN. She has a BA in Philosophy from Vanderbilt University (1998). She is a freelance photographer and graphic artist. In her spare time, Stacey enjoys playing badminton and documenting rural life in the U.S. and abroad.

Tom Wortham, a 1966 graduate of the University of Kentucky College of Pharmacy, is a resident of Madisonville, KY. Having recently retired from pharmacy, he now pursues his avid interest in photography.

Hand Drawn Artwork:

Taylor Politan, age nine, lives in Greenwood, IN. She would rather be outside than in; she loves all animals, especially reptiles, and she wants to be a veterinarian.

Hannah Cozzolino, age eleven, lives in Plainfield, IN. She loves softball and wants to be a hairstylist.

Morgan Cozzolino, age nine, lives in Plainfield, IN. She wants to be a pastry chef.

www.ingramcontent.com/pod-product-compliance
Lightning Source LLC
Chambersburg PA
CBHW061124070526
44584CB00033B/4212